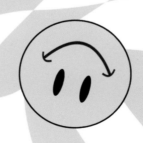

how not to fit in

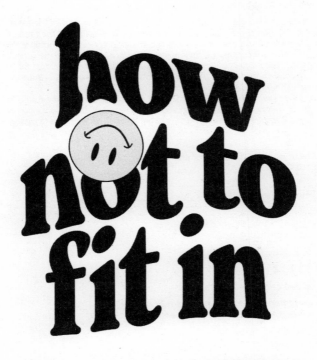

how not to fit in

An <u>unapologetic</u> guide to
navigating autism and ADHD

JESS JOY & CHARLOTTE MIA

Thorsons

Thorsons
An imprint of HarperCollins*Publishers*
1 London Bridge Street
London SE1 9GF

www.harpercollins.co.uk

HarperCollins*Publishers*
Macken House, 39/40 Mayor Street Upper
Dublin 1, D01 C9W8, Ireland

First published by Thorsons 2024

10 9 8 7 6 5 4 3 2 1

© Jess Joy and Charlotte Mia 2024

Jess Joy and Charlotte Mia asserts the moral right
to be identified as the authors of this work

A catalogue record of this book is
available from the British Library

HB ISBN 978-0-00-858922-6
PB ISBN 978-0-00-868702-1

Printed and bound in the UK using 100%
renewable electricity at CPI Group (UK) Ltd

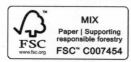

To Alix Burnard

An absolute ray of sunshine who was excited to read this book. Thank you for being the perfect example of how to live a life full of so much joy and meaning. Missing you endlessly.

Contents

Part 3: Navigating Neurodivergence

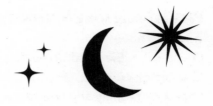

Introduction

Hi! Holy shit, you bought our book, thanks for that!

We're Jess and Mia, best friends and now business partners – who also happen to be neurodivergent. We created a now global online community back in late 2021 after realising that we were both autistic and had ADHD in our late twenties. And in a wild turn of events, we're now writing a book about the experience and our learnings so far!

We know that, particularly at the beginning, it can be traumatic to realise you're neurodivergent. Suddenly it makes sense **why** you've struggled with jobs, relationships, friendships … all the stuff that seems to come naturally to others around you. And with that comes the realisation that had you known about this earlier, perhaps life would've been easier. But as much as it can be tricky to have a brain like ours, it can also be a source of deep healing and joy.

Let us say upfront that we are still figuring all this out, only now, we have:

- ⚡ A lot less shame for what we're feeling
- ⚡ A better understanding of how to emotionally regulate ourselves
- ⚡ An ability to communicate our needs that we didn't have before
- ⚡ … and finally, a lot less desire to make ourselves uncomfortable for the sake of others

Living in a world that consistently tells you to be less of who you are can *understandably* mess with your confidence. But if either of our journeys so far have taught us anything, it's that knowing how your brain works, learning to resent it less and being a bit more aware of the standards you're holding yourself to makes it easier to walk around *without* feeling like you're tensing every muscle in your body. Not to reinforce the idea that it's all on us as neurodivergent people to execute all of the solutions or adjustments we need (because a world that is already adapted to how we work is the goal, right?) but being able to feel a little more in control and a lot more able to be less sorry about what works for us and what doesn't (when it's safe to, of course) can really help.

Historically, more men have been diagnosed with ADHD and/or autism than others, but we're now as a society learning that these types of brains (we'll sometimes refer to autism and ADHD as 'neurotypes') just show up differently in different people – a complete relief for those of us neglected by the outdated stereotypes. We'll talk more about self-diagnosis later in the book – but at the time of writing, it's estimated that one in seven people in the UK are neurodivergent (ND),[1] with most of those going undiagnosed. That said, the increase in awareness has led to more diagnoses, too. In the year ending March 2022, there was a 39 per cent rise in patients with an open referral for suspected autism, according to the NHS.[2]

The rise in interest and understanding of neurodivergence means there's new information and research about autism and ADHD being released all the time – and we seem to be finding out new things **constantly**. This book contains everything we know right now, but this is an ever-evolving journey.

In the course of writing this book, we've spoken to researchers and experts, but we're definitely not medical professionals and our views aren't static – they've changed and will continue to.

This book will elaborate on our (sometimes too) personal experiences with being autistic and ADHD, but because we all experience things differently (and because we are two white women who are, in many ways, very privileged) we've included the stories of many others, too.

Although we hope this book will appeal to anyone who identifies as neurodivergent or simply feels they can't quite fit in with the way the world 'expects' them to be, we'll be focusing on two labels specifically: autism and ADHD, as they are the ones we personally know best.

This Book Is for You If ...

⚡ **You're at the beginning of your journey.** Do you feel lost? Exhausted from feeling like you're stuck in the same old circle of trying and then failing (it's not failure, btw; navigating this world is **hard**)? Do you think, maybe, you might have a neurodivergent brain but don't know where to begin? We got you.

⚡ **You know you're neurodivergent** (whether you've self-diagnosed or a medical therapist has said so, both pathways are totally valid) and you just want to find a community. You're looking for people who get how you feel and can give advice on how to handle the tough situations life keeps throwing your way. Yep, we got you, too.

⚡ **You know someone who's struggling,** and you want to help them but you don't know how.

⚡ **You're interested.** Are you someone who's fascinated by the human mind? Do you want to know more about how others experience the world? You're in the right place.

How to Use This Book

POV: You've treated yourself to a shiny new book and you're entirely convinced that this WILL be the one you're finally able to read cover to cover.

We've got a revelation for you: this might not be that book (and possibly no book ever will be!), so let's instead just free ourselves of those expectations and run with whatever works for our brains without guilt, yes? If you struggle with focus, or if it takes you longer than other people to read, know that we get it.

Every ounce of this book has been written and designed for brains like ours. Want to start from the middle because it's a topic you're currently into, or scribble all over it or fold over the corners? No problem. Want to use it as a coaster so that it remains in sight and stands a chance of being picked up? We're here for it!

Throughout this book, you'll find:

- ⚡ Plenty of subheadings for context that will hopefully help you either stay interested or avoid what isn't of interest at the time.
- ⚡ Stories from us and other autistics and ADHDers.
- ⚡ Research and information from experts to help guide you further.
- ⚡ Space for your own journalling, jotting and processing (or even doodles if that's your kinda thing). At the end of each part, you'll find a discovery workbook where we'll prompt you to delve a little deeper into your journey.

If you're beginning to feel tired (or frankly just bored – no offence taken) after reading for what you consider 'not long enough', don't ignore it. Your way of doing things is not any less right than the way other people do things. It's perfectly fine for you to process things at your speed, and this book will still exist when your interest peaks again. Plenty of us know the 'shit, I'll put it down and never be able to pick it back up' feeling, but we're telling you right now to let go of that guilt. Throw that feeling out of the window for us, yes?

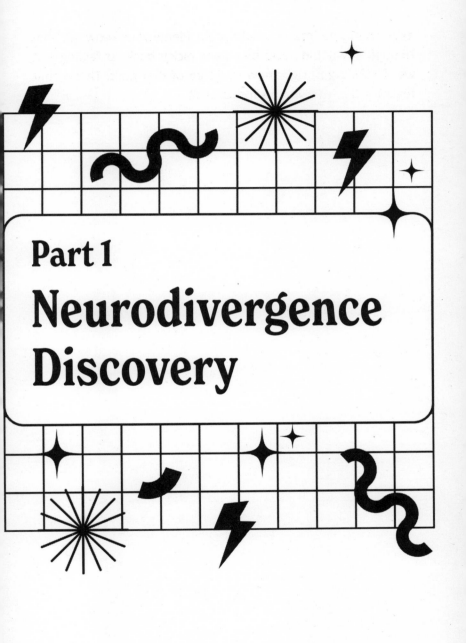

Part 1
Neurodivergence Discovery

Getting to Know Yourself

As you read this book, it's our hope that you get to know yourself and your brain better. We're aware that some of you might have picked it up with the smallest inkling that you don't 'fit in' somehow but have stopped short of delving any deeper – until now. Perhaps you're starting to realise that there are certain things you struggle with that others don't seem to. Maybe you're done with masking your true feelings, preferences and inclinations. When we felt completely lost and overwhelmed, we wondered why we couldn't manage as well as others and couldn't work out if we should squash those feelings and try to meet those standards, or create our own? Hell, we didn't even know if our experiences or traits were directly related to having spicy brains, or something else entirely. Connecting the dots between all of these things isn't easy.

All that is to say: the journey you're about to embark on might feel long, difficult and complicated, but be reassured that we've been there – and we run a community of over 100,000 others who are on this journey, too. In this first part, we're going to start by telling you our (very different) stories in the hope that a) they'll help you get to know just who's going to be talking to you for the next 350 pages and b) that you might see yourself in what we've been through. That said, we know our experiences can never reflect everyone's (how bizarre would that be?!), so while we kick off with our stories, you'll read those from many others as you make your way through this book.

And because we know some of you will be at the early stages of exploring what neurodivergence might look like for you, we're going to start at the very beginning, explaining what neurodivergence is and why it's being talked about so much at the moment. This is a huge subject to wade through on your own and we wouldn't have been able to do it without each other, so we're hoping that this book is your companion as you discover what all of this means for you. We'll explore what signs and traits are associated with ADHD and autism (outside of the generic and limited NHS lists you might have read online), how these might present, and why this expansion of understanding is a good thing (and long overdue). While it might not feel great all the time, this will be an affirming and rewarding journey – we promise.

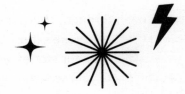

CHAPTER 1

Our Stories

⚡ **How we met**
⚡ **Where we are today**
⚡ **Founding I Am Paying Attention**

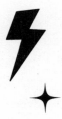

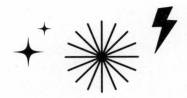

As this book is focusing on experiences (both ours and those of others), it's going to get cosy between us. We'll be constantly drawing on things that have happened to us throughout our lives so far – the good, the bad, the totally fucking disastrous – and what we've learnt from them. But first we wanted to give you a little synopsis of our individual journeys, as well as how we helped each other and how connecting with our bloody delightful community online has had a HUGE impact on our lives. So, if you'll indulge us ...

How We Met

We were 19, and probably too ready to grow up and begin living our very adult lives in Plymouth at university. If you believe in fate, you could say it stepped in and ensured that we'd both chosen to move to Plymouth, because that's clearly where all big dreams begin (that's sarcasm, by the way. No, we can't read sarcasm either). We were thrown together (along with a bunch of other students) into the accommodation building we affectionately called Disco Heights.

Neither of us can remember our **exact** meeting, as it was during Freshers' Week – that whirlwind time of running in and out of flats, meeting too many new people and generally feeling shit scared and out of place (but never admitting that to anyone). Within about a week of living in Disco Heights, we'd already become glued to each other's side. And in between occasional lectures and heavy drinking, we spent the next few years hiding in each other's rooms from the harsh reality of actually being at uni.

This was all before either of us knew we were neurodivergent. But, looking back, the signs were there. We both tried painfully hard to live the standard first-year-of-uni experience, but it was pretty obvious that we didn't enjoy it. We'd buy tickets for club nights, arrive and both eventually feel so overwhelmed that we'd either sneak off home together to sit and chat in one of our rooms, or take to the smoking area, where we'd find space (and air). Now, we'd have the language to say, 'I'm overstimulated here,' but back then we had to seek out other ways to feel even a little bit comfortable in (the many) situations we found awkward.

We planned quieter nights out to grungy pubs, where we could dress down and feel more like ourselves. It was a hard time for us both financially; we couldn't afford new outfits or to go out all the time like some of the people around us could. Instead, we'd go to Starbucks as a treat to try to make the best of a shitty situation. We were lucky to have each other, but the reality is that a lot of our time in Plymouth was **hard**. A huge amount of that was down to both of us not knowing we were neurodivergent. That big fucking truck was heading our way and would hit us in a decade's time. And it really **did** cause a lot of chaos ...

Jess

'Uh, what are we supposed to be doing again?!' Back when I was at school in the 2000s, my teachers were often completely oblivious to the fact that I'd stopped listening to what they were saying way before the task was set. I wasn't loud or disruptive, but staring out of the window or even just getting lost in my own thoughts, absorbed by whatever I was obsessed with at that time, was pretty standard for me. If I hadn't managed to find out from a friend, I'd quite often leave class wracked with anxiety, knowing that I'd been told what homework to do next but had zero idea what it actually was.

Despite this, my desperate need to please every person I came into contact with meant that I managed to get results that satisfied teachers – even if it meant sobbing in the early hours before a project was due to be handed in that I had forgotten about. Funnily enough, I didn't end up in detention once throughout my entire school career.

I had coping mechanisms before I realised they were coping mechanisms, and a support system that many people don't have access to. I'm super close to my mum – she's also (in my eyes) clearly autistic and, as a result, knew exactly how to validate and comfort me. Like me, she didn't know she was neurodivergent, but she's very self-aware and emotionally intelligent and knew instinctively what I needed. I'm eternally grateful for her support, but ironically I imagine it contributed to some of my struggles because it delayed me learning coping strategies for myself.

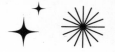

I didn't feel 'different' in the way I've heard so many people in our community talk about. I just felt … not enough. Consistently. I didn't know that the intense and overpowering feelings of anxiety were because I was always aiming for standards that just didn't fit with me or the way I needed to work. I was so wrung out with anxiety surrounding my GCSEs that I went to my GP to see if they could help. They didn't.

It felt like everyone around me was achieving and being successful, and generally managing to hold down a life **much** more easily than I was. I was baffled at how they were doing it. I was always left completely exhausted when I was trying to figure out where I was going wrong, and why what was being asked of me was so unattainable. I might be exaggerating slightly, but let me tell you, the amount of energy I find myself having to pour into many of my daily tasks and respon-sibilities has never seemed to align **at all** with what I see in my peers.

I remember having mostly male classmates who were 'naughty' and 'disruptive', displaying some of the stereotypical attributes associated with being autistic or ADHD, but they were nothing like me and, as far as I knew, I was nothing like them. I was the student who was sat next to those boys, in the hope that I would encourage them to focus. I couldn't see any similarities between us. Now, of course, I can see that I was masking (more on that in Chapter 6) and, in hindsight, I'm sure there are plenty of things that I have in common with them. But given that, as a society, the way autism and ADHD present in women and minorities has been at best misunderstood and at worst ignored, I was left to claw my way through every situation I was thrown into – then later, as an adult, to do the research myself with a shit ton of trauma to work through as well.

When it came to friendships in school, I was a bit of a 'floater', if you will. I'd drift between the different friendship groups, sometimes almost finding comfort and creating my identity around being 'different'. I also always took everything personally. There was – as in most high schools – a lot of drama, and according to my mum, I'd read into every tiny speck of my friends' body language, overanalysing and getting particularly upset by the tiniest of arguments. A combination of all the above meant that throughout high school my confidence was really low – I struggled to know why I found **everything** so difficult.

When I left high school I had this real need to escape the town where I grew up, so I went to college in Stourbridge, where my dad lives (my mum and dad split when I was three) to study art. Unfortunately, so did my boyfriend at the time. He was particularly shitty, which made finding the freedom I so desperately needed harder to come by. He also did nothing to help rebuild my shattered confidence. In fact, he made it worse.

When it came to university, I chose a place I was loosely familiar with (unfortunately because of said shitty ex), but otherwise Plymouth was a new place for me to roam around in as a relatively 'new' adult while I figured out what living alone was like for the first time.

In my first year I was living in Disco Heights with Mia, before we (along with another friend at the time) moved into a house together for our second year. Almost as soon as I arrived in

Plymouth, though, I began to dread the act of leaving wherever I was living and actually **going** to university. The problem? I know learning should be fun to some extent, but for me it was far from it.

When I first arrived I threw myself into it all – as much as I could: the house parties, the club nights where it was a pound a pint (I don't even drink beer), the pre-drinks where everyone scrawled over your T-shirt in felt-tip pens ... I was binge drinking (like everyone else), but alcohol is a depressant. **Not** good for a brain like mine. I also had no fucking idea how to navigate life and responsibility without the direction of an **actual** adult, so making it into uni consistently (and enjoying myself there) was a challenge, to put it mildly.

I found that I preferred sitting in my room in the dark or making my way into Mia's room to do pretty much the same (but with the addition of her company and fairy lights), to try to make my way through the huge lows I was experiencing. Second year came around, and on top of the mental discomfort, at some point I started experiencing some physical aches too. Just what I needed! The inflammation seemed to stay for days or weeks at a time before disappearing, only for another area of my body to experience the same thing shortly after.

This went on for months while I tried to make my way through another year of uni. All before my mum managed to convince me that this actually **wasn't** what I should be experiencing at 21. Plenty of blood tests and doctor's appointments later, I found myself crying in a hospital room after being told by a lovely consultant that I did in fact have lupus, an autoimmune disorder, which causes pain, swelling and discomfort in the body. Yes, I could take medication, but no, it wasn't going to go away. The perfect time to be entering my third year at uni weeks later, really. Particularly as Mia, by that point, had moved away from Plymouth, so I felt very alone.

It was a lot to deal with. I didn't want to be someone who had to take multiple tablets a day. I wanted to be able to eat freely without worrying whether it would leave me in pain for days afterwards. It was a grieving process. I had to leave behind who I was before. Third year was a horrid time, and it's a blur. But I managed to graduate, and although I knew I had some interest in business and marketing, I still hadn't found the direction I wanted to go in for work.

You might be unsurprised to hear that I went on to have many jobs – and a lot of struggles (and lessons) that came from them (we'll talk more about how to navigate wild workplaces in Chapter 10). After a rocky experience with my mental health over the years and never being able to find the reason why or any solutions, I was fired from the last job I had where I was employed by someone else. Many of the people in our community experience unemployment at higher rates than other parts of the population; and while I think we **do** get bored, feel unsatisfied, maybe even say things that other people deem inappropriate, or struggle with being on time, I also feel extremely strongly that there are things that are considered 'normal' in modern workplaces that are entirely unfriendly to neurodivergent brains and we, as employees, have very little power to change them. That's a huge part of why it's such an enormous fucking relief to be self-employed now, running I Am Paying Attention with Mia full-time.

I began to suspect I had ADHD in 2020 and got a clinical diagnosis in 2021 (we'll dive into diagnosis in Chapter 5). The realisation that I have autism as well followed. It brought me so much clarity, but also triggered a grieving process, because I realised that I'd spent so long thinking that I just wasn't good enough.

Where I am today

Now that I no longer have to bend, and struggle, and change myself to fit into a school or work environment, I've managed to find so many different and actually quite exciting ways to make work **work** for me. I've also been in a happy, supportive and healthy relationship for five years with my partner, Ryan, who I live with in Warwickshire with our dog, Leo. Life today, though never perfect, looks pretty good, actually.

'I feel grateful every single day to be best friends with someone who, despite whatever life is throwing at them, is always able to show kindness, patience and understanding. The fact that you've managed to reach a point of peace and happiness in your life makes me so happy because I can't think of anyone that deserves it more than you.' – **Mia**

Mia

Like so many, I didn't pursue a diagnosis or even have suspicions that I was autistic or had ADHD until I hit a point of total breakdown in my life. I had experienced a fair few setbacks, but every time I thought I had reached rock bottom, it turned out another fucking rock was waiting for me. So I guess the easiest way for me to tell you my story is by revisiting each of those rocks …

Rock one

'If you carry on the way you're going, you'll end up stacking shelves in Tesco' were the words I heard from the head of my university course. I was 19. I remember just sitting there, stunned. I'd gone in to see him to get some direction, positive that he might be able to help me. He'd asked me where I saw myself in five years' time and I'd smiled and said, 'In a graphic design role' – it was what I was studying, after all – and he'd **laughed** before making that gross and classist remark. It also began a large spiral of shame and diminishing self-esteem.

In summary, I failed university catastrophically.

Three things you expect from uni: education, friends and a degree.

The three things I got from uni: **mental illness, shame and debt**.

While I did have some very supportive tutors, not knowing how to communicate the help I needed robbed me of getting the education I wanted. I often wonder how different my experience would be if I went to university now, knowing what I know about myself and the way I work.

Rock two

Back home in Bath, in my early twenties, I knew I **had** to make something work, so I launched myself into applying for jobs while trying to build a portfolio for myself without a degree. I probably worked four times as hard as I would have if I'd actually got my degree, and for that very reason I managed to launch a career for myself in the design agency world.

The only problem was, I lacked a lot of the technical skills required to keep those jobs. In the design world you need to be well skilled in various design programmes. I was creative and ambitious, but I had a lot of catching up to do. I was self-teaching, and so I struggled to keep up, as there was so much I needed to learn. I was also way too ashamed to admit that I was so far behind my co-workers, so I kept quiet, squirrelling away in the evenings and at weekends, exhausting myself in the process.

I worked myself to burnout. Not just **once**; I was in a constant cycle of burnout.

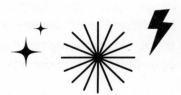

It usually went:

ambition > work myself into fight-or-flight mode > performance slips > struggle to keep up > get fired > fight-or-flight mode > end up in the same position and repeat.

I continued this cycle for nearly 10 years. Not only was my nervous system a complete wreck, but I was so riddled with shame and low confidence from constantly feeling as if I was letting myself down that I began to fall out of love with design. Maybe I just wasn't that good at what I did. No one else seemed to struggle like I did. Why did it often feel like I was doing life on Level: Hard? After I lost three or four jobs because I was struggling, I felt like I had really hit rock bottom and I wasn't sure where to turn. But guess what? It was **not** rock bottom ...

Rocks three, four, five and six

I've always known exactly what to do to get a job and develop healthy relationship habits. At first. My struggle is how to maintain them. For several years I managed to find routine and structure again – I managed to hold down a job, a relationship and even move cities. Life felt vaguely manageable.

After lots of rejections I landed a design job in Bath, for an **actual** company with an office. It wasn't exactly the type of design I saw myself doing, but at this point I was just happy to have found some stability and I managed to hold it down long enough to gain some real experience – until I inevitably got fired again (this time for poor attendance). But I was so used to things going this way that it wasn't even a shock. I had a little cry, found another job and then decided I wanted to move to Brighton. So, along with my partner at the time, I moved to Brighton, found a new design job with real responsibility and a salary that meant I could actually afford to live. Things were looking up.

It probably won't come as a shock when I tell you that soon enough the shit hit the fan. This time it was ACTUALLY rock bottom, as it wasn't long before I was back into my cycle – over-working to burnout, not being able to communicate what was wrong and getting fired. I struggle with memories, particularly from traumatic moments in my life, so it's been really hard to recall what happened during this time, but I lost everything in that period of my life. The person I was for the next year or so is now completely unrecognisable to me; it was a brutal mix of no stability, no job and frankly an inability to hold down a healthy relationship.

I was running, big time – and although I didn't know then exactly what I was running from, I knew my nervous system was in fight-or-flight mode for well over a year, and I'm not sure any words I'll ever throw together will quite scratch the surface of how awful it was to live through the day to day.

Where I am today

I eventually managed to get subsidised therapy and it was my therapist who helped me realise that I had struggled so much because I am autistic and have ADHD, and I'd been struggling to fit into a world that wasn't suited to me.

The reality of juggling adult life means that we don't always have the capacity to process things that need to be processed, especially not all at once – and if I've learnt anything from the journey Jess and I have been on so far, it's that this shit takes time to work through. As much as I'd like to be 'out the other side', I'm still not there yet – rather, I'm just trying to be gentle with myself and live peacefully while I make my way through it. But I can say I'm in a happy relationship, working with my best friend **and** sharing my story with you to showcase that no one is alone.

'It is mind-blowing to me that someone can have so many obstacles thrown at them and still consistently find a way to be authentically herself. Having a best friend (and now business partner) who is so keen to learn how to be softer in a world that makes it hard to do so, who knows all the right moments to pull out dark humour (and all the right moments to be delicate), is one of the things I am most grateful for every single day.' - **Jess**

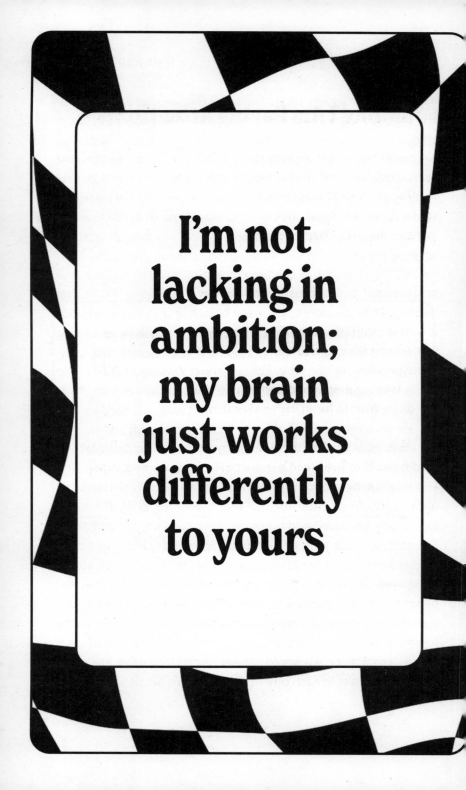

Founding I Am Paying Attention

A common question we get asked is, 'When were you diagnosed with ADHD/autism?' And while we totally recognise that getting an official medical diagnosis is important and life-changing for some, for others it may not be necessary (we'll delve into all this in more detail in Chapter 5).

For us, the moment of change came not because of a medical professional, but because of **ourselves**. This happened during the COVID-19 pandemic; we were both trapped inside without any of the coping mechanisms we might usually have access to (like having structure to our days!) and it became a time of deep introspection. While we'd always known we were similar in many ways, we also had something else in common: we both fitted the criteria for ADHD and autism.

We were both stuck in this seemingly never-ending cycle, where we'd be able to live life in a manageable way, holding down jobs and relationships, but the effort of doing so in a world that didn't understand us or cater for our brains was huge. We'd end up exhausted, confused and burnt out from working so hard. We'd inevitably lose our jobs, or a relationship would splinter, and then we'd feel like we were back at square one again. We knew something **had** to change. So, as we're both overly self-reflective people who, like many who are autistic and have ADHD, can spend hours studying and getting to know our topics, we slowly began to recognise ourselves in tweets and others' individual stories. From there, we would have endlessly long iMessage chats recognising traits in each other that aligned to ADHD and autism.

While both of us had experience with medical professionals, it was the support of each other, and the validation that came with it, that made the biggest difference. All our lives we'd had people tell us that we were 'exaggerating' or dismiss us when we tried to be vocal about how and why we found the world hard. So we really needed each other to say, 'No, that's not right, **you shouldn't have to try this hard**.'

The topic of conversations went from 'Can you write this email for me because I physically cannot do words and I'm terrified of the recipient hating me?' to 'Big ADHD energy' and 'That sounds a lot like something an autistic person would say' – sometimes those three topics might even be discussed within a single iMessage conversation (if you know, you know).

There were plenty of times when we're not sure we'd have managed to keep ourselves going without the cheerleading and support from the other. Even if that sometimes looked like us taking the piss out of how awful things felt – because no matter how depressed and financially screwed you are, apparently dark humour always makes things better if it's coming from your best friend. We wanted that for others. Which is how our baby brand and business, I Am Paying Attention, was born.

We realised that there were undoubtedly a lot of people out there like us, experiencing the same things but without the safe, cosy, judgement-free friendship we had in each other.

It all came out in one phone call. A huge long one involving so many tears, but also a lot of BIG realisations. It was that conversation that made us realise, 'Wait a minute, if we are feeling like this, how on earth is anyone coping with this who doesn't have a best friend constantly in their pocket?'

Inspired by the reassuring words we'd throw at each other because we were fidgeting or looking elsewhere while psycho-analysing ourselves over FaceTime, Mia created the I Am Paying Attention Instagram account at the start of November 2020 – a place for us to dump some of the reflections we'd been working through.

Boldly sharing the parts of us we'd felt ashamed of and had kept hidden for so long was a cathartic process – and it turned out there were a lot of people who were navigating life while nursing the same gnarly wounds.

Growing our community

We'd initially enjoyed the idea of other people benefiting from our work, but it was **entirely** beyond what we expected when we started receiving hundreds of messages from people telling us they'd sobbed while scrolling through our feed, or that we'd introduced them to the idea that they **weren't** just 'not working hard enough'; in fact, their needs weren't being catered to in everyday society.

To this day, we still receive plenty of messages that leave **us** with watery eyes – and so, without disclosing anyone's painfully vulnerable feelings, instead we'll tell you that those messages collectively prove that there are so many people like us, people with ADHD and autism, who have gone – and **still are** going – **far too long without the support they need and deserve**.

Of course, it feels good to have your efforts appreciated, but it's also a very bleak realisation that an Instagram page is the closest thing to validation and resources that thousands of people have. Sure, there's information out there, but as we discovered before setting up this account, most of that information is, ironically, formatted in a way we couldn't really process – or, most importantly, wasn't speaking to people like **us**. It was usually aimed at the parents of young children, often with a not-so-subtle undertone of 'get your child to behave better and inconvenience you less' – or they were spouting utter shit like 'autism is less common in girls'. Once we've read something we know to be wrong, we're probably not going to trust anything else it's saying. Right?

We realised that, like us, a lot of the adults who were following us needed validation, some practical tools and alternative approaches, a reminder that they deserve respect as they are and, above all, a community to assure them they're not alone.

Our healing conversations over text were redesigned by Mia to become our social media content – and although that was a complex thing to navigate in itself (apparently 24/7 deep conversations aren't always good for your brain either), we managed to create a space where we'd realise that the way we'd been forced to do things up until this point didn't work for many of us, and there actually **were** ways of doing things that didn't neglect our needs.

Accessibility

Just as we've done with this book, we also took a lot of time to think about what made our content accessible or inaccessible (and while we're very much aware that accessibility doesn't start and end with brains like ours, we also felt as though our community deserved to be able to absorb our content with ease, you know?). Here are a few golden rules we came up with:

- ⚡ **Support shouldn't be full of jargon,** formal language and designs that don't work for our brains. As we started to realise that the way we've been expected to process information for the entirety of our lives has only contributed to the setbacks we've faced, it became even more important that we got this right.
- ⚡ **Use examples wherever we can** – because we were speaking to people who had been shamed for not being able to retain bits of information, or to fully grasp points that were being made, unless there were examples.
- ⚡ **No pages full of text.** As our audience were people like us, whose brains would nearly always lose interest when they saw a page full of text, we had to give them our thoughts in a way they'd be able to benefit from. We've tried to do the same in this book, and break text up, or at least try and make it look a little more dynamic.
- ⚡ **Watch out for visual stress.** We'd have conversations with people who reminded us that visual stress is often something autistics and ADHDers experience, and we made changes off the back of their feedback. We'd try to find the balance between 'interesting enough to catch the

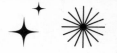

eye of an ADHDer' and 'not so overwhelmingly bright that it will physically pain those who are also dyslexic'.

Who is our audience?

When we first began, there were plenty of comments from delightful (privileged) men. They were getting pretty riled up whenever we spoke of the difficulties we associated with not knowing how we worked – or rather, not having the language to describe it until later in life – because our experiences (as autistic women who also have ADHD) didn't reflect theirs. It was like they felt that by sharing our experiences, we were taking something away from them.

You know what's ironic about that? As we'll come on to in Chapter 5, men are also the people whose symptoms are most accurately reflected in past versions of the diagnostic criteria. We're all too aware that displaying characteristics associated with autism or ADHD – whoever you are – can mean you're on the receiving end of unfair treatment and ableist comments, but the repeated harsh words we were receiving from men whose neurodivergence is commonly represented left us sitting with the reality of how hard it is to be someone who is left behind.

Not only did nobody see our struggles as they were happening, but once we'd managed to connect the dots ourselves, we were reminded that not everyone was going to believe us.

We'd like to say that the shit from them only fuelled our fire, but that would be partly lying. It pissed us off, and it was utterly exhausting to be putting everything we had into healing our pain (and allowing strangers on the internet in on the very raw, vulnerable journey), only to have to find more energy from somewhere to advocate for ourselves.

'Ignore them!' people said. That's all well and good, but we're traumatised, remember?! The thought of not being liked by everyone pulled up a lot of Big Old Feelings about consistently not being enough, but it was an uncomfortable reality we involuntarily worked through – because we sure as shit weren't going back to a traditional nine-to-five job.

With time, we figured that these particular types of commenters could be presented with a whole feed full of information or long responses explaining our reasoning, and they'd still feel as though our experiences were somehow worth less airtime than theirs. So, we decided to focus on sharing our own experiences in the hope that they resonated with others like us. We had to learn to block those dudes out.

From the very beginning of this passion-project-turned-job, we wanted to hold space for many of the people whose struggles have been ignored and show what neurodiversity **really** looks like. At the time of writing, we have over 100,000 followers (come and join us over at @iampayingattention). Later on, we will be speaking to some of the wonderful people we've met through our community, and online, to ensure that we're giving voices to as many people as we possibly can.

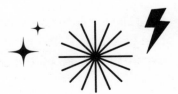

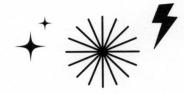

CHAPTER 2

What Is Neurodivergence?

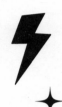

⚡ **Examples of neurodiversity**
⚡ **The link between ADHD and autism**
⚡ **Labels and autism**

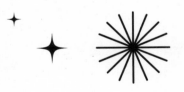

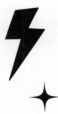

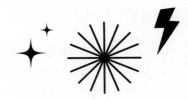

We're going to spend some time exploring the language in our community, how it's used and how we feel it has helped and/or hindered us. And where better to begin than with the umbrella term 'neurodivergence'?

Coined more than two decades ago, neurodivergence describes the idea that ...

> **'People experience and interact with the world around them in many different ways; there is no one "right" way of thinking, learning, and behaving, and differences are not viewed as deficits.'[1]**
> – Harvard Health Publishing

Some examples of neurodiversity include ADHD, autism, dyslexia, dyscalculia, dyspraxia and Tourette's syndrome. As we have experience of ADHD and autism, this book will mostly explore those two conditions, but below is a summary of what each of these terms means:

- **Autism:** According to the National Autistic Society, autism is a lifelong developmental disability that affects how people communicate and interact with the world. In the UK, official figures indicate there are about 700,000 people on the autism spectrum.[2]
- **ADHD:** The NHS defines attention deficit hyperactivity disorder (ADHD) as 'a condition that affects people's

behaviour. People with ADHD can seem restless, may
have trouble concentrating and may act on impulse.'[3] In
the UK, according to the National Institute for Health and
Care Excellence, the prevalence in ADHD in adults is
estimated at 3–4 per cent.[4]

⚡ **Dyslexia:** A common learning difficulty that mainly causes
problems with reading, writing and spelling.

⚡ **Dyscalculia:** A learning difficulty that affects the ability to
use and acquire mathematical skills.

⚡ **Dyspraxia:** Also known as developmental co-ordination
disorder (DCD), this is a condition affecting physical
co-ordination. It can show itself in children when they
perform less well than expected for their age in daily
activities and appear to move clumsily.

⚡ **Tourette's syndrome:** A condition that causes a person
to make involuntary sounds and movements, which are
referred to as tics.

If you want to learn more about what neurodivergence means
in its full glory, we recommend checking out the work of brilliant
public speaker, advocate and author Sonny Jane Wise (@livedex-
perienceeducator).

WTF Is 'Neurotypical'?

Neurodivergence describes a brain that diverges in any way
from the typical – or the neurotypical. But what is a typical
brain? While there are significant developmental differences in
neurodivergent brains, we find ourselves thinking more and
more that the idea of a 'neurotypical' brain is actually a load of

shit. Some people believe that neurotypical isn't a type of person, but more a set of oppressive standards, moulded by capitalism.

Microbiologist and writer Dr Ayesha Khan, who goes by the handle @wokescientist on Instagram and writes a Substack of the same name, speaks of this concept in their Substack piece 'Yes, we're all a little neurodivergent'.[5] They say: 'No one is biologically wired to thrive under capitalism and a lifetime of being socialized with oppressive norms harms everyone. Just because someone is able to conform, doesn't mean they enjoy it or are "built" for it. Some are able to conform better than others because they have more privilege or some have to conform as much as possible because their severe marginalization leaves them no choice.' Perhaps, therefore, a 'neurotypical' person could just be someone with a brain that is better able to conform to society's capitalist expectations.

The Link Between ADHD and Autism

Although there are some known risk factors that can increase the likelihood of developing autism and ADHD, nobody really knows what causes these conditions. What we do know is that there is a lot of overlap between their symptoms. 'There is some crossover between neurodiversity traits,' explains Leanne Cooper-Brown, neurodevelopmental clinical lead at Clinical Partners, one of the UK's leading mental health, autism, and ADHD services, who has over 20 years of experience working with autistic people. 'For example, most neurodiverse conditions impact what we call "executive functioning" [more on this on pages 54 and 289], which means people have trouble with things like problem solving, planning and keeping track of tasks. Sensory issues are also seen across different neurodiverse conditions.'

Leanne points out that while this can make diagnosis difficult, each condition does have a clear set of criteria with traits that are exclusive to each. 'This helps us differentiate between them,' she says. As for the crossover between ADHD and autism, Leanne explains that some ADHD symptoms may look similar to autistic behaviours. 'For example, we see limited reciprocity [responding to the actions of another person] in both, but the reasons can differ. A person with ADHD may struggle with conversations due to distractibility whereas someone with autism may struggle with conversations due to difficulties reading social cues.'

There are a lot of people in our community (Jess included) who only started exploring autism after furiously researching ADHD. This is partly to do with the overlapping symptoms, but also partly due to the increased social stigma of autism compared with ADHD. What do we mean by that? Well, a lot of the ways that autism can present (such as being non-speaking) are things that many people are made to feel ashamed of. There's nothing wrong with non-speaking communication, but again, because our world is built around neurotypical ideals, autism has been used against these types of people in the past. Whereas for ADHDers a lot of the traits surrounding it, such as being late or not managing to focus, can be perceived as charming, or even cute (patronising, much?), even though, as we know, they can also land you in a lot of shit. So we can see why the journey to an autism realisation might begin with ADHD, as it's (slightly) more accepted in our society.

High- and Low-functioning Labels and Autism

First of all, let's unpack what these terms have traditionally been used to mean. 'High-functioning autism' isn't an official medical term or diagnosis; it's used by some in the community (though others totally disagree with using the term) to talk about an autistic person who can speak, read and handle basic life skills such as eating and getting dressed. Essentially, they can live independently. Someone with 'low-functioning autism', on the other hand, is usually unable to live independently and will need help from a guardian throughout their lives. The definition of autism has changed so much over the decades, and most likely will again as we learn more, but the high/low labels are often used by people who argue that the spectrum is too broad and that someone with 24-hour-care needs can't be compared to those of us who live independently.

'Oh, so you **must** be a high-functioning autistic, right?' Believe us, besties, we hear this a lot. It's frustrating as the person saying it is making an assumption based on the person standing in front of them – they can see that we're put-together, in a nice outfit, smiling and chatting, but they can't see what's going on underneath all that and how much effort it took to get there.

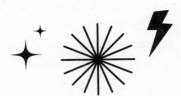

This is one of the (many) reasons why the high- and low-functioning labels used to really piss us off. It's why we, and many others in our community, choose **not** to use the terms. They reduce us to what others see, rather than encapsulate what we're actually experiencing – and for those of us who've only managed to get through life because we've hidden our true selves, our struggles don't feel 'mild' or 'less severe', which seems to be the assumption that comes with the high-functioning label when we disclose that we're autistic. It's unfair to say that those of us who manage to hold down jobs are 'high-functioning' and others, who (as an example) are non-speaking, are 'low functioning'. Neither one of those people are worth more than the other, and both are equally autistic.

We do understand, though, why some people might like to use these labels. In fact, we absolutely believe that anyone within the community should be able to use whichever set of labels makes their life easier, saves them energy or represents who they feel they are on the inside. After all, if someone wants to describe themselves as low-functioning then they absolutely should: perhaps to them – to you – that term means your autism is non-verbal, and using the 'low-functioning' label is helpful when it comes to explaining it. We think, though, that there's nothing wrong with being non-verbal. It's another way of communicating. We shouldn't be pushed to see our ways of living and surviving in this world as flaws. A lot of the criteria as to whether you're a high- or low-functioning autistic person is down to how you function in **this** society. How would you see yourself if you were functioning in a world that actually catered to your needs? When it comes to conversations surrounding autism and ADHD, a lot is pinned on how well you can perform to meet society's expectations. We might **look like** we're managing, but that doesn't mean that we're not burning out as a result of doing so, that we're able to wash or feed ourselves independently (and yes, prompts and reminders count as support), that we're able to navigate life without the support of another person, or that we're able to communicate when it's expected of us.

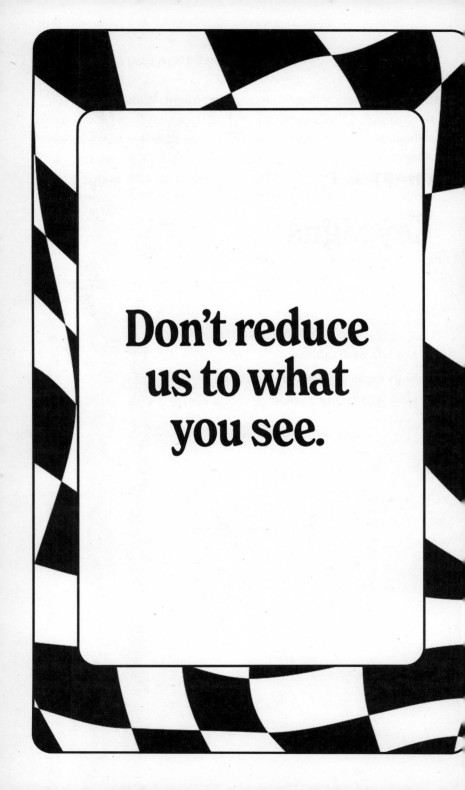

Don't reduce
us to what
you see.

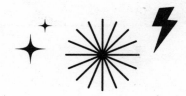

CHAPTER 3

Key Signs

⚡ **Models of disability**
⚡ **Keys signs of ADHD and autism**
⚡ **How ADHD and autism show up for us**

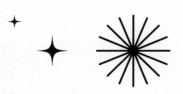

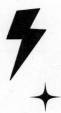

We slowly began to figure out that we could be autistic ADHDers not from a medical professional or journal, but from **real** people talking about their **real** experiences online. In a way that gave us hope, that told us, 'No, it's not that you haven't found the right time-management app, you probably struggle with this stuff for a reason.' These people framed experiences we could recognise in a way we'd never considered before. It was phenomenal. And that's why we want to keep sharing our own experiences.

But before we get into the details about the specifics of how neurodivergence 'looks', we need to start with a bit of a disclaimer – and if you've ever read our Instagram captions, you'll know we absolutely love a disclaimer. Why? Because this shit is complicated. As anyone who has found themselves lost within medical jargon or been dismissed by a professional knows, **the research in this area has a lot of catching up to do when it comes to reflecting everyone's experiences of ADHD and autism**.

We don't want to contribute to any further misinformation, and we know that for each and every one of you your journey will be different. We want you to be able to see yourselves, but our experience will be different from yours, which is why we are harnessing the power of our community and the research that we trust.

In an ideal world, this is where we would include a long list of autism and ADHD symptoms and you would tick them all and be certain that's you, right? **The reality is that ADHD and autism show up differently in every person.** Although there are quite a few similarities regarding focus or sensory sensitivities, there are also a lot of variations in how we actually experience these things.

For example, two people could read an article headlined 'Do you hate the sensation of sex? Then you could be autistic' – person A could be left thinking they're autistic, and person B could be left thinking they aren't. In reality, they could both be autistic (or not). Truthfully, some of the spiciest women we've ever met are autistic – and the point we're making is that there is **such** a wide range of experiences out there that, as Leanne Cooper-Brown explained on page 39, it can often be tricky to pinpoint the defining characteristics of these conditions.

The key signs can look very different from person to person, and for many reasons. Perhaps you grew up in a household where a lot of neurodivergent traits were picked up on or even criticised, without the person understanding that the trait is associated with neurodivergence. Did you struggle with remembering homework due dates? Did you struggle when things weren't routine at home? Perhaps family gatherings were especially taxing. A lot of these things can just be considered rude by others, so you end up absorbing those messages and thinking you're just 'difficult' or 'lazy'. You can twist yourself into knots thinking, 'If only I had more discipline,' or, 'If only I was more like this person,' when you're trying to fit yourself into a model that wasn't designed for you. So it's important to remember that you're **not** all those nasty things you tell yourself. You just have a different way of being.

The medical model of disability has been the absolute standard within psychiatry and psychology for at least the past few hundred years holds that autism and ADHD are disorders with symptoms. We don't like this. We don't think we have a disease that needs curing. While we use labels like 'attention deficit hyperactivity disorder' and 'autism spectrum disorder', we firmly believe there is nothing **disordered** about us. Later in this chapter, we'll explore a different model of disability that better fits how we see ourselves.

There are many valuable conversations happening within the community about how certain labels or terms like these might be perpetuating ideas that we're lacking or broken in some way. But still, those terms are a reminder that for a large part of history, people have failed to understand that there are several ways of functioning in the world around us, and no single one of them is superior.

There **may** be certain people who manage **somehow** to better fit a society that demands consistent energy levels and productivity from us, and there are also many things people with brains like ours have going for us – and if we're brutally honest, our value doesn't lie in those traits either. We, and you, are enough as we are, whether we struggle to manage daily life in a capitalist society or not.

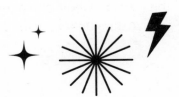

All that being said, we can see that it's useful to have some sense of what the common signs and traits of ADHD and autism can be, so let's take a closer look.

ADHD Traits

The NHS says that the symptoms of attention deficit hyperactivity disorder (ADHD) can present themselves in three forms: inattentiveness, hyperactivity and combined.[1]

Most people with ADHD have challenges that fall into these categories, but this is not always the case, and some people's traits change significantly over time through each life stage.

For example, some people with the condition may have challenges with inattentiveness, but not with hyperactivity or impulsiveness, and might instead better fit the criteria for attention deficit disorder (ADD).

These are some of the traits that the NHS say can be signs of ADHD[2]:

- ⚡ You get easily distracted and find it hard to notice details, particularly with things you find boring.
- ⚡ It's hard to listen to other people – you may find yourself finishing their sentences for them or interrupting them.
- ⚡ It's hard to follow instructions.
- ⚡ You find it hard to organise yourself – you start a lot of things without ever finishing them.
- ⚡ You find it hard to wait.

- ⚡ You fidget and can't sit still when there's nothing much going on.
- ⚡ You're forgetful and tend to lose or misplace things.
- ⚡ You easily get irritable, impatient or frustrated and lose your temper quickly.
- ⚡ You feel restless or edgy, have difficulty turning your thoughts off.
- ⚡ You find stress hard to handle.
- ⚡ You tend to do things on the spur of the moment, without thinking, which gets you into trouble.

Autistic Traits

According to the NHS, the below list encapsulates the common signs of autism in adults:[3]

- ⚡ Finding it hard to understand what others are thinking or feeling.
- ⚡ Getting very anxious about social situations.
- ⚡ Finding it hard to make friends or preferring to be on your own.
- ⚡ Seeming blunt, rude or not interested in others without meaning to.
- ⚡ Finding it hard to say how you feel.
- ⚡ Taking things very literally – sarcasm could be really hard to understand.
- ⚡ Having the same routine every day and getting very anxious if it changes.

You may also have other signs, such as:

⚡ Not understanding social 'rules', such as not talking over people.

⚡ Avoiding eye contact.

⚡ Getting too close to other people, or getting very upset if someone touches or gets too close to you.

⚡ Noticing small details, patterns, smells or sounds that others do not.

⚡ Having a very keen interest in certain subjects or activities.

⚡ Liking to plan things carefully before doing them.

Autism can sometimes present differently in women and men. Autistic women may:

⚡ Have learnt to hide signs of autism to 'fit in', by copying people who don't have autism.

⚡ Be quieter and hide their feelings.

⚡ Appear to cope better than autistic men with social situations.

⚡ Show fewer signs of repetitive behaviours.

Thinking Outside the Box

The lists we've just given show the 'official' traits associated with ADHD and autism according to the NHS, but in recent years (now that research on both has expanded to include more diverse groups of people), we're learning that the signs of these conditions go far beyond these limiting lists. 'The criteria is outdated and very gender defined, because the majority of the research was carried out on young boys. This results in women being left behind, as well as adult males,' says Pauline Harley, a career and self-advocacy coach who runs a women's peer support group with a National Autism Charity in Ireland, and was diagnosed as autistic herself aged 45.

'Psychologists are currently working on getting it to be updated with the new traits that are coming through as more people talk about and discuss how neurodiversity displays in them. It's important to discuss the different traits and how, although there's common ground in all autistic people, we all display traits differently. There could be one person who is not bothered by sensory stimuli and another for whom it causes a panic attack.'

As Harley says, psychologists are learning about new traits based on the experiences they're hearing about from people like us. You might find that ADHD and autism show up as struggles with:

- Dealing with mail.
- Changes of plans.
- Closing containers/ cabinets.
- Basic self-care.
- Booking appointments.
- Answering questions on the spot.
- Recalling information.
- Cleaning out the fridge.
- Decision-making.
- Waking up.
- Negative self-talk.
- Remembering passwords.
- Controlling emotions.
- Focus and being easily distracted.
- Regularly making little mistakes.
- Worrying about being fired.
- Getting bored easily.
- Leaving clothes in the washer.
- Losing your keys.
- Being productive at 2 a.m.
- Hot drinks going cold.
- Taking criticism personally.
- Feeling like you are lazy.

- ⚡ Lacking motivation.
- ⚡ Irritability.
- ⚡ Detachment.
- ⚡ Frequent mood swings.
- ⚡ Daytime sleepiness.
- ⚡ Forgetting verbal instructions.
- ⚡ Leaving things to the last minute.
- ⚡ Forgetting to eat.
- ⚡ Zoning out during conversation.
- ⚡ Overly emotional.
- ⚡ Feeling defensive.
- ⚡ Being uncomfortable in clothing.
- ⚡ Monotropism (see below).
- ⚡ Stimming (see opposite).

What is Monotropism?

A monotropic mind is one that focuses its attention on a small number of interests at any one time, tending to miss things outside of that attention tunnel. Monotropism is thought by some to be the central feature of an autistic brain. It's also our comfort-blanket state – one we often revert to when facing or in the midst of burnout. The problem? It means we focus on one thing and then forget everything else, resulting in a prolonged period of unmet needs. For example, a polytropic mind might answer the question, 'How are you?' with a broad overview of what they're up to and how they feel, whereas a monotropic mind will give you an extensive monologue or essay on their deepest thoughts and desires. We often find ourselves thinking, 'How can I possibly get across everything that I'm feeling right now?' – and that's our monotropic minds in action.

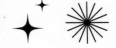

What is Stimming?

According to the National Autistic Society (NAS), 'stimming' or 'self-stimulating' behaviour includes 'arm- or hand-flapping, finger-flicking, rocking, jumping, spinning or twirling, head-banging and complex body movements'. They also say 'it includes the repetitive use of an object, such as flicking a rubber band or twirling a piece of string, or repetitive activities involving the senses (such as repeatedly feeling a particular texture)'. Obvs, that's all very medical and you might have other stimming behaviours that you don't recognise on this list. Jess calls the way she twiddles her fingers her 'sparkly hands', and she loves to twiddle with her hair. It's basically behaviour that makes you feel soothed, and the NAS also add that 'stimming doesn't necessarily mean you are autistic or have ADHD, but it is a common trait in neurodivergent people'.[4]

Executive Dysfunction

Many ADHD traits are symptoms of executive dysfunction. That's not us going all corporate on you (would we ever?), but an actual medical term. 'So, what does it mean?' we hear you ask.

Well, executive functions are cognitive skills such as being able to pay attention, regulate emotions and multitask. On the flip side, executive dysfunction describes not being able to do these things. You know, when you're in freeze mode – you have so many things you need to do but you just **can't** do them.

Executive dysfunction is common in people with ADHD, and also in those with brain damage or diseases that affect the brain.

Pre-realisation, we didn't know why this was. Then, post-realisation, we had this **word** for it and, yep, it describes exactly what we're experiencing. Executive dysfunction isn't just a case of lacking motivation. Nor is it this cute, ditzy thing. It has real impact. We'll talk more about how it shows up in our lives in Chapter 14, but, for example, we once left important life admin for so long that it cost us a lot of money. It can also mean not being able to shower, or brush our teeth. Discovering the term 'executive dysfunction' helped us understand our brains and has been an important part of our journey.

What Does All That Look Like in Real Life?

It's true to say that we've experienced most of these traits at some point. At times we studied them, memorised them and applied them to every single aspect of our lives. But we don't do that anymore. Why?

- ⚡ It was incredibly traumatising to spend so much time thinking how life could have been different had we realised we were 'neurodivergent' earlier (we can't change the past, ffs).
- ⚡ A lot of these things are part of the human experience. We can't pathologise our entire existence.

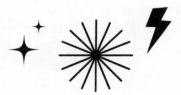

But that doesn't mean it's okay when people turn around and say, 'Oh, you don't like doing your washing? **Nobody** does – stop looking for an excuse not to do the hard things in life.'

After all, it's not like we just sit back and get everyone to do everything for us. We **do** the hard things, the tough things, and it takes us so much effort and is so exhausting. Which is why, at the beginning of our journeys, examining the traits – and how they applied to our lives – was vital. It helped us explain to people (when we needed to, as we shouldn't have to educate **all** the time) why we struggled with some things more than others.

Are We Disabled?

The diagnostic criteria for ADHD and autism are commonly framed to highlight how much of a burden you are to neurotypical society. Earlier, we mentioned the medical model of disability. As a reminder, it says people are disabled by their impairments or differences. According to the medical model, these impairments or differences should be 'fixed' or changed by treatments, even when the impairment doesn't cause pain or illness. To us, that suggests we are the ones lacking in something. That we are disordered. That we are broken. That the fact that we can't perform certain things well is essentially **our** fault.

BUT!

The social model of disability says that disability is caused by the way society is organised, rather than by a person's impairment or difference, and was developed by disabled people, activists and sociologists in the 1970s in the US. It looks at ways of removing barriers that restrict life choices for disabled people and focuses on YOU – the disabled person – and how society's narrow view of how things should be has effectively disabled you. As disability charity Scope UK says, 'Barriers can be physical, like buildings not having accessible toilets. Or they can be caused by people's attitudes to difference, like assuming disabled people can't do certain things.'[5] This we love. It's telling us that we are disabled by the lack of accommodation for us in society. By the obstacles that society puts in place. We are not lacking, we just have a different way of being and the world doesn't cater to that, which makes navigating life much trickier.

The problem? While the social model of disability makes total sense and was created by disabled people themselves, we've grown up in a world that is shaped around the medical model that says we need to be fixed. If we hadn't grown up in that world then maybe, just maybe, we wouldn't feel like our traits disabled us. Basically, we wouldn't feel like we were broken.

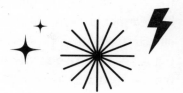

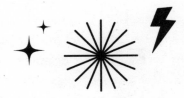

CHAPTER 4

Why Are Autism and ADHD So Underdiagnosed?

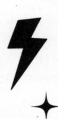

⚡ **The research on diagnosis**

⚡ **The impact of underdiagnosis**

⚡ **Why is underdiagnosis happening?**

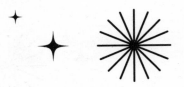

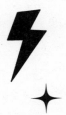

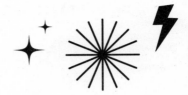

Let's kick this off by saying outright that underdiagnosis isn't just a women's issue: it's a sexism, racism and classism issue. Although recent headlines have focused on the underdiagnosis in women, those who are also affected by it include the trans community, people from minority ethnic backgrounds, and young boys who don't fit the heteronormative standards. Basically, anyone who doesn't slot into the category of young white male who presents as hyperactive has historically not been accounted for in the research on ADHD and autism, and therefore is likely to fall into the group of people who have gone undiagnosed.

What the Research on Autism Tells Us

Don't get us wrong, it can be mega-comforting seeing the proof that there are others out there like you in a cold, hard statistic. To look at a percentage of the population and realise, 'Hey, I'm not alone!' We get that. But, just so you know, when it comes to the statistics, often these studies have been carried out with a neurotypical lens, or have used surveying criteria that hasn't quite caught up with the conversation online (e.g. a question could involve listing a bunch of ADHD/autism traits that aren't recognisable to you, as they don't relate to your existence as a woman or a minority), so the numbers could still be a little skewed or higher than those you see overleaf. With that said, below are a few of the latest stats and findings regarding autism diagnosis:

- ⚡ The number of patients in March 2022 with an open referral for suspected autism in the UK was **103, 215**. This is an increase of **39 per cent** compared with the year before. Oh, and of the patients with an open referral, **84,625** had referrals that had been open for at least **13 weeks**. Autism referrals have tripled since 2019 and waiting times have **quadrupled**.[1]
- ⚡ Boys are **four times** more likely to be diagnosed with autism than girls.[2]
- ⚡ In 2021, most children were being diagnosed after the **age of four**, although autism can be reliably diagnosed as early as **age two**.[3]
- ⚡ Autism affects **all ethnic and socioeconomic groups**, yet minority groups tend to be diagnosed later and less often.[4]
- ⚡ ADHD affects an estimated **30–61 per cent** of autistic children.[5]
- ⚡ Nearly **80 per cent** of autistic women are misdiagnosed, often with other conditions such as borderline personality disorder, eating disorders, bipolar disorder and anxiety. It's currently unknown how often women with ADHD are misdiagnosed.[6]
- ⚡ Autistic girls and women may go **undiagnosed** because doctors, teachers and even parents often think of the condition as primarily affecting boys.[7]
- ⚡ A reported trait is that females might be **more likely** than males to '**mask**' their autism features by mimicking their non-autistic peers.[8]

⚡ According to research by LGBTQ crisis support service the Trevor Project, **transgender boys/men and non-binary youth** report the highest rates of suspecting they may be autistic, but have relatively low rates of diagnosis.[9]

What About ADHD Research?

And below are some stats and findings from the latest research on ADHD:

⚡ According to consultant psychiatrist Dr Rob Baskind, speaking in **Forbes** magazine, the percentage of individuals with ADHD who are treated is 10-20 per cent.[10]

⚡ The percentage of adults who have ADHD but do not know it is **75 per cent**, according to Len Adler MD, a leading researcher in adult ADHD and a professor of psychiatry at New York University.

⚡ According to studies that look at who meets the ADHD criteria in the global population as a whole, the ratio of boys to girls with suspected ADHD could be anywhere between **2:1** and **10:1**.[11]

⚡ Research suggests that girls need to have more severe, and more visible, symptoms than boys before their ADHD will be recognised. One study of 283 children aged between 7 and 12 years old looked at what differentiated both boys and girls who met the diagnostic criteria for ADHD from those who had a lot of ADHD symptoms, but not enough to be diagnosed. It was found that parents, in their own ratings, seemed to **play down girls' hyperactive and impulsive symptoms**, while playing up those of boys. They also found that girls who did meet the criteria tended to have **more emotional or behavioural problems** than girls who didn't. This was not the case for boys.[12]

⚡ In a similar study of 19,804 Swedish twins published last year, it was discovered that girls, but not boys, were **more likely to be diagnosed** if they suffered from hyperactivity, impulsivity and behavioural problems.[13]

⚡ In 2013, after surveying more than 17,000 US children, it was found that by the time the study's subjects reached eighth grade (that's 13 to 14 years old) **African American children** were **69 per cent** less likely – and **Latino children 50 per cent** less likely – to receive an ADHD diagnosis than their white counterparts. A follow-up study, in 2014, found that the disparity actually started earlier: before they even entered kindergarten (so nursery), African American children were **70 per cent** less likely to be diagnosed with ADHD than white children.[14]

So, What's Going On?

It's now obvious that just because more boys are **diagnosed** as autistic and ADHD, that doesn't necessarily mean more boys **have** autism and ADHD. The stats show that women and non-binary badasses are more likely to go undiagnosed, so why is this happening?

The fact is that determining how autism and ADHD present in us can actually be pretty complex. Many of us have relied on extensive coping mechanisms and 'masking' techniques (more on masking in Chapter 6) to get by and blend in, but it doesn't mean we don't have autism and/or ADHD, nor does it mean we're not struggling. That's why it's so important to have a full picture of how ADHD or autistic traits can show up, as we discussed in Chapter 3.

Given that a large percentage of us have literally had to 'cope' in order to survive, we're finding that a lot of us **are** actually able to do a lot of the things in the criteria that those with ADHD and autism are supposed to find difficult. That **doesn't** mean, however, that we do that easily. For most of us, it takes a huge amount of effort, at the hardest level, leaving us with little to no energy as a result.

Perhaps this is why women and non-binary people often receive a diagnosis of depression, anxiety and borderline personality disorder before an ADHD diagnosis (because who feels good about themselves when they're struggling to do everything required of them day to day?) – and that can only further compli-cate the diagnosis journey.[15]

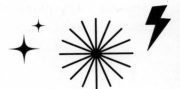

Rebecca's Story

Rebecca, 20, is studying law and in her final year at university and was diagnosed with ADHD in 2022. She is currently pursuing an autism diagnosis.

When I look back on my childhood there were so many opportunities when my ADHD and autism could have been picked up on. But my family, like many Black families, ignored anything to do with mental health. I was even, at one point, offered therapy and when they found out they stopped me from going. I was also placed, in primary school, in a special support group for kids struggling with socialising. But they pulled me out of that as well. I remember being sad at the time, as it had been helping.

I'm a smart person. I don't struggle academically, but I do struggle with focus. When I receive the support I need I perform really well. In secondary school my English teacher always took the time to sit and support me when I needed. And because of her I absolutely loved English and I was good at it. But the other teachers didn't recognise this. If I didn't do well, they'd just try to throw me off the course.

There was one teacher – a nasty man who was known to be racist to other non-white pupils – who stands out in my memory. I was in Year Nine and I'd found a way to sit on chairs that was comfortable to me. I'd sit sideways and let my legs hang off the arm rests. He kept me after class and when I tried to explain to him that sitting in the 'standard' way physically caused me pain, he screamed in my face. His spit landed on my cheek. I left in floods of tears. I couldn't breathe. It was my first ever panic attack.

I'd see other kids who, when they displayed 'obvious' signs of ADHD, were offered support. There were the boys who were disruptive, and even white girls who were quiet or introspective. Often I think whenever I showed signs I'd just be stereotyped – like I was behaving how they expected Black girls to behave.

I've recently received my ADHD diagnosis thanks to I Am Paying Attention, who did a video on other routes I could go down.[16] I was on a long NHS waiting list and they said I could go via Psychiatry UK, so I did. [**Note from Jess and Mia:** We'll talk more about this route in Chapter 5.] My diagnosis has helped me so much. It's given me access to university support – everything from my lecturers giving me more time, to grants and additional software, which helps. I've also learnt to be kinder to myself post-diagnosis. I sometimes worry I'm overstepping the mark when it comes to seeking support. I know that's my internalised ableism, which I'm working hard to deconstruct. I did similar work a few years ago to deconstruct my internalised racism, but this is a whole other ball game. It's a lot to process.

I received my diagnosis just as I was entering my second year and, looking back to my first year … I was just running around like a headless chicken. Now I make sure to take regular breaks, go for walks and runs every day and take my studying slowly. With law there's so much reading, so it's essential I don't get overwhelmed. My diagnosis has also meant I am now on medication. If, for whatever reason, I skip a day and don't take it

I can notice myself slipping back into old habits – like not sleeping or eating.

From my own research I'd always known I was an ADHDer, but family stigma meant I couldn't pursue a diagnosis until I was 18. This has been one of the major barriers in getting my autism diagnosis – they need someone to vouch for me who knew me when I was younger. But my family won't do that. One of my biggest fears is them finding out about the process and putting a stop to it. I also don't have any friends from when I was younger as I struggled to make them, so it's a real issue.

I've gone through a lot of grief, thinking what could have been if I'd had access to the support I needed earlier. I've shown how much potential I have when the world caters to my needs. I know I'm doing well, but I really think I could have succeeded so much more. I could have been the first Black woman on the moon! But there's still time …

Hey! This Is All Terrifying: The Impact of Underdiagnosis

Besties, if you're in a tough place right now, consider skipping this bit – for now – as we're about to get real. The impact that underdiagnosis and the stereotypes associated with ADHD and autism have on real, beautiful, wonderful people like you is difficult to process, so reading on may be triggering. Take care of yourself, first and always.

'The lost generation' – that's what researchers at Edge Hill University in the UK called the significant number of adults who received a late diagnosis for autism.[17] Many of them reported a poorer quality of life and mental health issues as a result of it. But why? As Leanne Cooper-Brown of mental healthcare practice Clinical Partners says: 'Autistic people and those with ADHD have to live in a world that is catered for neurotypical people.' (Amen, Leanne!) 'They have to expend much more energy to manage daily tasks that come naturally to non-neurodivergent people. This can lead to anxiety and fatigue. In addition, neuro-diverse people have sensory differences that impact their emotional regulation.'

The Edge Hill study surveyed 420 autistic and typically developing adults, and interviewed eight autistic people who were diagnosed late in adulthood.[18] The reasons for the late diagnoses probably won't surprise you – parents not wanting to pursue a diagnosis because they had bad perceptions of autism came up, while those with lower support needs, who were therefore considered 'high-functioning', tended to slip through the cracks.

We know the huge impact poor mental health can have – we both still suffer from deep, dark bouts of depression – and the stats on this are terrifying. According to research and campaigning charity Autistica, autistic adults are nine times more likely than non-autistic adults to die by suicide,[19] while in 2022 the Trevor Project said that young LGBTQ+ people who had been diagnosed as autistic had 'over 50 per cent greater odds of attempting suicide in the past year compared to those who had never been diagnosed as autistic'.[20] While, of course, everyone's

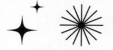

mental health is individual and it's not known what factors contribute to suicide in each case, those at Autistica have been told by sufferers that delays in diagnosis, difficulty accessing support and poor physical health have contributed to their feelings.[21] For those in a minority group who are already facing discrimination, this can feel like a pile-on of problems, especially as autistics and ADHDers are more likely to suffer from anxiety and depression.

Relationships repeatedly breaking up and breaking down, being fired from jobs, self-medicating with drugs and alcohol ... You're probably already aware of how living with undiagnosed trauma – whether because of your neurodivergence or for another reason – can be truly shit.

And there's a phenomenal amount of research backing up the fact that navigating life while desperately trying to fit in, or being told you're **wrong**, has a hugely detrimental effect on mental health and wellbeing (not that we need research to validate what we already know, but sometimes it's useful). Research carried out in 2015 on the importance of getting an ADHD diagnosis showed that undiagnosed ADHDers had poorer relationships, both personally and professionally, leading to lower self-esteem (we're citing the study here, but, of course, we believe you don't need an 'official' diagnosis to know you have ADHD).[22] There's also a link between ADHD in childhood and partner violence,[23] as well as an increase in alcohol and substance abuse.[24] Gah! Is it any wonder we struggle with these conditions being ignored/unrecognised when it can lead to so many other issues?

If you're struggling with suicidal thoughts or ideation, there's help out there, and there are so many people on your side. You can reach the Samaritans on 116 123.

White Privilege and Autism

We're both very aware that we are approaching our journeys through the lens of white privilege. Everything from our ability to look deeper into how to unmask, and why and how we mask, to how much energy we expend trying to meet neurotypical standards is influenced by our own white privilege. Black and brown people, alongside those from other marginalised communities, not only have to meet neurotypical standards; they have to do so while also dealing with racism and a whole host of other issues. It's a huge, huge topic and one that we don't have direct lived experience of, so we want to use our platform to highlight the works of people we have learnt a great deal from.

One of these was an incredible article, written by Morénike Giwa Onaiwu, entitled '"They Don't Know, Don't Show, or Don't Care": Autism's White Privilege Problem', in which she highlights how the portrayal of autistic characters in television and other places (as mostly white and male) deeply and terrifyingly impacts people of colour. She points out that it wasn't recognised in the cases of Arnaldo Rios, Reginald 'Levi' Latson, JT Torres, Kayleb Moon-Robinson or David Ramos – all autistic individuals of colour who were unjustly (and, in most instances, violently) mistreated by US police officers. She writes:

In all of these cases, the intervening officers perceived these individuals' mannerisms as aggression rather than character-istics of autism and responded with excessive force. Although the officers' actions are clearly reprehensible, it begs the question: with such little recognition that autistic people of colour even exist, should we truly be shocked by any of these incidents? Or by the recent deaths of Eyad Hallaq of Jerusalem or Elijah McCain of Colorado, both young men of colour who displayed autistic characteristics and were killed by the police?[25]

She argues that 'society at large, particularly those who are more privileged – are uninformed of the realities of those whose lives are more laden with oppression than theirs', but also that there are those who could make a difference (working within the medical industry) that aren't. She asks 'allies, families, fellow autistic people, etc. of all ages, genders, races, and backgrounds' to 'continuously increase your knowledge of matters relevant to autism and race',[26] in order to begin the work desperately needed. These examples sound extreme, but as we learnt from Rebecca earlier in this chapter (see page 66), race can play a significant role in how easily – or not – a person of colour can access a diagnosis and/or the support they need.

Cultural factors also play a huge role, as we learnt when Kaiomi Inniss, a Black Caribbean woman with ADHD, wrote a piece for us on how, in the Caribbean, many people she loves and knows dismiss mental health issues, with (she writes) 'some parents viewing their children's disabilities as a parenting failure'.[27] It's why she struggled to get her diagnosis and still struggles to get her parents to accept her ADHD. But, she explains, 'I do not blame my parents for not noticing or believing; our broader cultural and societal dynamics reinforce negative ideas about people with disabilities'. Throughout her journey she has been angry that, as a Black woman, she's had to advocate so hard for herself in the medical system, and this is something we have come across so many times in the articles we have read and from the people we have spoken to.

Why Are So Many People Being Diagnosed with ADHD and Autism Right Now?

Did you know that from the 1800s to the 1960s, people were discriminated against for being left-handed? School kids were **forced** to write with their right hand, and many languages still contain references that conflate left-handedness with stupidity and dishonesty! It's wild. But then, in the early 1970s, acceptance of the fact that being left-handed is totally normal and natural began to grow. People spoke about being left-handed, and guess what? The number of left-handed people shot up.

This wasn't because **suddenly** way more people were being born left-handed. It was simply because people felt less ashamed to speak up about being left-handed and stopped pretending to be right-handed. So couldn't the same thing be happening today with ADHD and autism? As the statistics we included earlier in this chapter show, between April 2021 and March 2022, there was a 39 per cent increase in open autism referrals.[28] But we don't think (as some ass hats seem to) that these numbers indicate an 'over-diagnosis' problem. Hello?! Is it not obvious from all the research that the opposite is the case, and that instead more and more previously underdiagnosed groups are having their very valid traits recognised?

Even though women, non-binary people and others from marginalised communities have been neglected by the scientific research community for decades, things **are** changing. There are more people with ADHD and autism working in the scientific fields than ever before (guess what? Our traits make us very good at research), and there are also many of us now being open about our experiences online and showcasing that ADHD and autism display themselves differently in different people. This means that, just like when we had our realisation in 2020, more people are recognising themselves in others' experiences, and feeling less shame (and there should be no shame AT ALL) in coming forward and saying, 'Yep, I'm an autistic ADHDer.'

Over the past few years there have been so many conversations and so much new research surrounding neurodiversity. We absolutely love this! Particularly as they highlight the experiences of women, non-binary people and others previously left behind. When we first began our journey it felt as if ADHD and autism traits took up our entire personality, and as if our realisations of how they impacted on us made up the majority of our conversations. It was constantly: 'Oh my God, look at this! Have you read this?' Slowly we've learnt that while being women with ADHD and autism does make up a large part of who we are, and impacts many areas of our lives, it doesn't define our entire personalities. We really hope that pulling these things apart in these chapters and the workbook you're about to read helps you navigate your self-discovery and how to meet your needs.

The Part 1 Workbook
Neurodivergence Discovery

Chapter 1: Our Stories

1. Now that you've heard our stories, think about your
    personal experience. Did you have a lightbulb moment
    where you realised you were neurodivergent?

    ....

    ....

    ....

2. Looking back, have there been any moments in your
    life when you felt you were held to unfair standards or
    misunderstood? In friendships? At work or school?
    At home?

    ....

    ....

    ....

3. Reflecting on your journey, are you still in the thick of it? Do you feel like you have a pretty good handle on things right now? Is there anything you feel like you'd kinda like to leave behind or move past?

....

....

....

4. Do you feel like you know yourself well right now? Or do you think there's a lot left to uncover and you don't know where to turn? (Been there!)

....

....

....

Chapter 2: What Is Neurodivergence?

1. Are there any neurotypical standards that you find difficult to navigate? Example: The expectation that everyone can hold eye contact comfortably (like in job interviews – in what world is it normal to stare at a total stranger right in the eyeballs for an hour?!).

....

....

....

2. How do you feel the stereotypical representation of autism or ADHD affects how you view your own experience? Example: If you mask (see Chapter 6) heavily, do you feel like your autism or ADHD is less valid because people (unfairly) expect more of you?

....

....

....

3. Do you ever feel discouraged by the media's coverage of ADHD and autism becoming a trend or being overdiagnosed? Example: Many of us can't access medical diagnosis straight away, nor do we always want to – maybe media coverage might make you feel as though your struggles are an overreaction?

....

....

....

Chapter 3: Key Signs

1. What was your 'it all makes sense now' moment? Did you even have one? Was there anything in particular that made you think, 'That sounds way too much like me for it to be a coincidence?' Example: Learning about monotropism (see page 54).

   ....

   ....

   ....

2. How has working through this process impacted your self-confidence? Example: Has it boosted it? Has it done the opposite? Or has it been a combination of both at different times?

   ....

3. In which area of your life (work, relationships, friendships) do you feel being neurodivergent affects you the most?

   ....

   ....

   ....

4. Which parts of your brain and personality are you learning to appreciate the most? Example: How exceptionally creative you are or how passionate you are about the things you're interested in, or maybe even that you see details that so many people miss.

    ....

    ....

    ....

5. Do you feel like there are any neurodivergent 'traits' that you don't relate to? Example: An immediately obvious struggle with social situations.

    ....

    ....

    ....

How this shows up for you personally

As you dive deeper, you might start to notice that you experience certain traits more than others – and while this might feel potentially inconvenient, it'll actually help you get to know how to adjust to your surroundings, maybe communicate your needs with the people around you, or even help you inform your medical practitioner, if that's a route you want to take. Part 2 of the book is about really understanding how these traits impact your day-to-day life. What specific things do you personally experience? We've included our list from Chapter 3 here, but feel free to scribble down your personal experiences as they happen.

- Dealing with mail
- Changes of plans
- Closing containers/ cabinets
- Basic self-car
- Booking appointments
- Answering questions on the spot
- Recalling information
- Cleaning out the fridge
- Decision making
- Waking up
- Negative self-talk
- Remembering passwords
- Controlling emotions
- Focus and being easily distracted
- Regularly making little mistakes
- Worrying about being fired
- Getting bored easily
- Leaving clothes in the washer
- Losing your keys
- Being productive at 2 a.m
- Hot drinks going cold
- Taking criticism personally
- Feeling like you are lazy
- Lacking motivation
- Irritability
- Detachment
- Frequent mood swings
- Daytime sleepiness
- Forgetting verbal instructions

☐ Leaving things to the last minute

☐ Forgetting to eat

☐ Zoning out during conversation

☐ Overly emotional

☐ Feeling defensive

☐ Being uncomfortable in clothing

☐ Monotropism

☐ Stimming

Chapter 4: Why Are Autism and ADHD So Underdiagnosed?

1. If you're someone who's late-realised or diagnosed, when you look back to when you were younger are there any clear signs that make you think, 'Someone probably should have picked up on that'? Example: Regularly covering your ears to block out sound, or your inability to focus in lessons.

....

....

....

2. Do you have any underlying frustrations about why nobody picked up on your struggles related to neurodivergence, which you maybe haven't sat with yet? (This isn't a place where you need to dial down your anger – let that shit out.)

....

....

....

3. Let's be real: not knowing this information until later in life is tough. Have you had conversations with anyone about it? Do you feel like there's anyone who might be able to relate to what you're going through (online or in person)? Example: My sister hasn't necessarily had the same experiences, but I think her insight into my childhood makes her a really good person to vent to about it all.

....

....

....

4. What do you think the younger version of yourself might need to hear?

    ....

    ....

    ....

5. Do you think you suppressed any part of yourself because nobody recognised (or acknowledged) your neurodivergence?

    ....

    ....

    ....

6. Given that so many of us are now realising that ADHD and autism look different in everyone, there are plenty of people questioning the rising rates of diagnosis. If you're hit with an opinion that goes something like, 'Wow, everyone seems to have ADHD and autism these days!' it can be a little ... enraging! It feels good to have an idea about what points you might want to bring up. List a few of yours (they might be from this book!) here.

    ⚡ ....

    ⚡ ....

    ⚡ ....

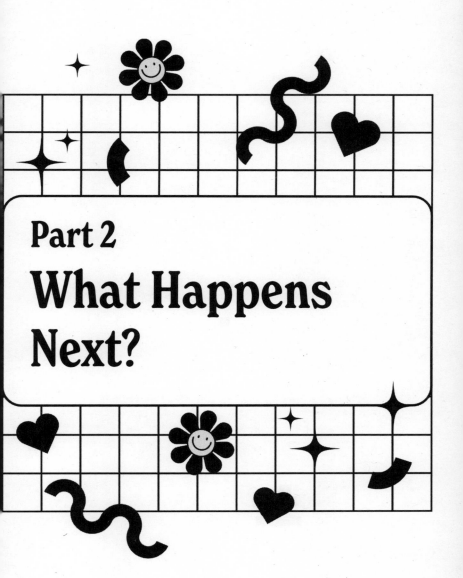

Part 2
What Happens Next?

Handling the Hard Stuff

Warning: You might be about to dig into some pretty tough stuff, if you haven't already. In this part, we're going to be trying to answer some of the questions that might be arising for you now that you've got to know your brain in a bit more detail.

You might be pulling on some interesting strings that you maybe haven't before; you might be looking at past experiences through a different lens and feeling more curious about whether you have autism or ADHD, or both, if you haven't got a self-identified or clinical diagnosis already.

Once you've done some of this introspective work, you might have more questions than answers and – we're going to be real with you here – it might feel worse before it feels better (but better is coming, we promise). These situations can vary so much for all of us: we're all different people with entirely different lives and experiences and traits, so there's no one-size-fits-all, step-by-step guide that will magically provide clear-cut solutions for you.

There's a lot to think about: what about diagnoses? What if you're not sure where to turn next? How much of yourself should you reveal, and at what pace? How can you handle some of the (probably pretty big) emotions that come up as you navigate this process?

A lot might come up for you, but remember, **your traits aren't deficits, even if society has made you feel like they are**. So much of what we feel about ourselves – especially the bad stuff; the stuff we've buried – is dictated by social norms, and the ways in which society values some things above others. Although it will be painful at times, this journey is also about reframing and rejecting some of the conditioning you'll undoubtedly have experienced as an ND person trying to make their way in a neurotypical world.

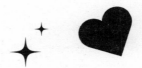

CHAPTER 5

Do You Need a Diagnosis?

⚡ **The diagnosis process**
⚡ **The validity of self-diagnosis**

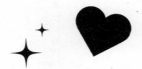

Are you thinking about whether you could be autistic or have ADHD but are worried about whether you are overthinking it? Maybe you're scared of being told you aren't neurodivergent because it'll invalidate how you feel about yourself (yes, we've had those 'If I'm not neurodivergent then I'm just a fuck-up, right?' thoughts before).

Well, we say that these are a good sign that you should look into it. The actual process of learning about neurodivergence, and how different all our brains really are, is very freeing. Pursuing a clinical diagnosis might be part of that journey for you, and let us say from the top that whether you do or not is completely up to you, and will entirely depend on your unique situation.

The diagnostic process can be difficult for many reasons, but the main issues are that it requires you to drag up years of potentially painful experiences, and that the actual process itself is entirely non-neurodivergent-friendly. Think you have ADHD? You'll need to fill out form after form, have multiple phone calls and probably chase your GP over a series of months because you haven't heard back (because you are on a waiting list – a waiting list that might be months, or even years, long).

You see our point? That's why, as we discussed in the previous section, we place more emphasis on your own 'realisation' – aka the moment **you** realise you have autism or ADHD. For many, this is a more meaningful turning point. Equally, though, having a diagnosis can give you access to certain benefits, as well as helping you feel secure when talking to loved ones about ADHD and autism.

Benefits of an Official Diagnosis:

⚡ It may help you and your friends and family understand ADHD and autism better, and what steps and coping techniques you can all put in place to make life easier.

⚡ It may help correct a previous misdiagnosis.

⚡ It may help you get better access to benefits, medication and appropriate services.

⚡ Your employer, school or university has to help you and make adjustments.

Okay, So What Are Medical Professionals Looking For?

According to the NHS, below is what happens during an autism assessment.[1] For children, the assessment team may:

⚡ Ask you about your child's development, such as when they started talking.

⚡ Watch how you and your child interact, and how your child plays. **[N.B. A girl might have learnt to play in the way that's 'expected' of her.]**

⚡ Read any reports sent by their GP, nursery or school. **[Studies have shown that teachers' knowledge of**

autism usually comes from the behaviour most commonly displayed in boys.][2]

⚡ Ask about their medical history and do a physical examination. A member of the team may also visit your child's school to watch them in class and at breaktime.

For adults, the assessment team may:

⚡ Ask you to fill in a questionnaire about yourself and any problems you have. **[This might feel traumatic to fill in. It's common to have a block and do everything you can to avoid doing this!]**

⚡ Speak to someone who knew you as a child to find out about your childhood. **[But what if you're estranged from your family?!]**

⚡ Read any reports from your GP about other health problems you may have.[3]

According to the NHS,[4] below is what happens during an ADHD assessment for adults:

⚡ The specialist will ask about your present symptoms. However, under current diagnostic guidelines, a diagnosis of ADHD in adults cannot be confirmed unless your symptoms have been present from childhood. **Again, what if you're estranged from your family? Or what if you learned to expertly mask your traits as a child?**

⚡ If you find it difficult to remember whether you had problems as a child, your specialist may wish to see your old school records, or talk to your parents, teachers or anyone else who knew you well when you were a child.

⚡ Look for symptoms which also have a moderate effect on different areas of your life, such as: underachieving at work or in education, driving dangerously, experiencing difficulty making or keeping friends, or experiencing difficulty in relationships with partners. **What if you made friends with people who were also neurodivergent? Or if you have ADHD and are autistic, your need for structure and predictability might have masked your hyperactive traits.**

'I diagnose autism and ADHD – this is what it's like'

We asked Leanne Cooper-Brown, the neurodevelopmental clinical lead at Clinical Partners, one of the UK's leading mental health, autism, and ADHD services, about how she goes about diagnosing and what the shortcomings are that she faces ...

How is autism/ADHD currently diagnosed?

With autism, the gold standard is to use a standardised developmental history such as the ADI-R (Autism Diagnostic Interview – Revised) or DISCO (Diagnostic Interview Social and Communication Disorders) alongside clinical observations and the ADOS (Autism Diagnostic Observation Schedule). Different clinicians of different disciplines should carry out both assessments. We also use supplementary questionnaires for children to gather school information. Once all the information is gathered, the clinicians will meet as part of a multidisciplinary team and review the information against the diagnostic criteria (ICD10 or DSM5) to formulate a diagnosis or non-diagnosis. The clinician will then give feedback on the outcome to the patient.

With ADHD, again a developmental history is gathered as well as a clinical observation. Tools such as the Conners (a rating scale and questionnaire about a person's behaviour, social life and work) are completed by parents and schools and the DIVA (Diagnostic Interview for ADHD in adults) can be used for adults. Again, the ICD10 or DSM5 can be used to determine if someone meets the criteria.

What are the difficulties you face when trying to diagnose autism/ADHD?

Difficulties include not having a clear developmental history, as both conditions are lifelong and pervasive, so we need to identify that traits were apparent in childhood. This is especially difficult in older patients where we may not have a caregiver informant. Also, if a person has experienced trauma, they may develop similar traits to autism, which can be difficult to differentiate.

There's been some criticism of the research and diagnostic criteria being outdated. Do you think this is true?

As clinicians, it is important we keep up to date with new research and literature which informs our clinical practice. I think there is definitely room for revisions to the current tools from research about how modern living impacts behaviours and social interactions. We would also benefit from tools more sensitive to the different presentations of autism and ADHD that we are now aware of.

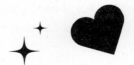

Jess on ... her ADHD diagnosis

Do you feel that having a diagnosis will make everything magically easier? Or that it'll help you feel at peace and move forward confidently into life with a label that makes sense of things? I did, too! Except it didn't quite work out that way. And, funnily enough, it doesn't work like that for most of the neurodivergent people I've met either.

A couple of years ago I was **all** about a medical diagnosis. I was pushing for one, but navigating all the forms and communication was **so** hard for me. So, as we've already discussed, I now think the focus should be on the moment of **realisation**, rather than being given the equivalent of a shiny green sticker from your doctor that proclaims, 'I HAVE AUTISM AND ADHD!' Having a brain like this is normal. So many people have a brain like mine. The world not being built to accommodate my brain is what makes things hard, **not** me.

But it's taken me a while to get here. Over the last couple of years, since learning about ADHD, autism and the finer details of my own brain, my relationship with labels has changed several times. I feel very strongly that we should **absolutely** use whatever terms feel comfiest to us.

I first began to recognise that my brain was a little spicy when I had a few super-emotional outbursts in response to things like noises coming from the TV or eating sounds. They resulted in me sobbing and slamming doors. At the time I couldn't understand why I was reacting so strongly, but now I know that those things were causing me genuine sensory distress. I was keen to figure out what was going on. When I headed to Google to describe my experiences, things like 'highly sensitive person' came up. I distinctly remember seeing ADHD mentioned along the way, so I began to follow ADHD people on social media who were discussing their experiences.

Many months later, being sure I had ADHD, I still felt like I wasn't able to use that label online. Because I didn't have a clinical diagnosis, I thought there might be people who called me out for 'making it up'. So I went through the official process and **finally** I was equipped with the ADHD diagnosis that I thought was going to be the answer to everything. I now knew that reactions I'd previously been ashamed of (like sobbing and slamming doors when the TV had been too loud) were because of sensory overload, not because I was being overdramatic. My shame at these 'overreactions' was compounded by the fact that other people's perceptions of these behaviours is gendered – generally, girls are socialised to be quiet and compliant, whereas the same isn't expected of boys. Even 'overreactions' in neurodivergent boys aren't viewed the same way as those displayed by neurodivergent girls. The diagnosis gave me some clarity, but I was still struggling – we'll come onto why later in this chapter.

How About Medication?

First, we'd like to say upfront: there's nothing wrong with you. We don't think you need a 'cure' for your wonderful neurodivergent brain. As we mentioned earlier, we believe in the social model of disability, which states that we shouldn't have to change; it's the expectations of the society around us, which are making us disabled, that should change.

When it comes to autism, there is currently no medication available, and the NHS are warning people to watch out for fake treatments that can be harmful.[5] Basically, anything that a) has cost you a lot of money and isn't on the NHS or b) claims to be a 'miracle' cure for autism is probably fake. Your doctor may suggest approaches you can take to make living with your autism easier, but they should **never** suggest medication.

There is, however, medication that's suitable for ADHD. There are five medicines available on the NHS, and while they're keen to stress that these aren't permanent cures (and again, we don't really like terms like 'cure' as they imply there's something wrong with you), they can help you concentrate better, and feel calmer and less impulsive.

Jess on ... medication

In 2021 I was in a cycle of not being able to function. I was regularly experiencing serious bouts of sobbing and feeling inadequate, as though I wasn't coping. I already had a prescription for ADHD medication but had been putting off taking it.

As I was struggling so much, I decided to try the medication and, at first, it blew me away. Tasks that before had seemed insurmountable were suddenly possible. Mia and others around me said there was a noticeable difference in me. It allowed me to approach tasks without feeling hugely overwhelmed.

However, I have a complicated relationship with food (which I'll discuss more in Chapter 13) and when I was younger I would obsessively monitor my weight. I've done a lot of work to cultivate a healthier relationship with food; I have removed bathroom scales from my life, and I no longer look at calories. But the medication suppressed my appetite and took the joy out of eating for me. I felt that if I continued to take it, I risked slipping back into my old eating habits.

So, I decided to stop taking it. I haven't taken it in a while and who knows? Maybe I will go back to it at some point, but as I've now got a toolbox of strategies for managing my ADHD, I feel okay not relying on it each day.

Niamh's Story

Niamh, 28, from Dublin, Ireland, was diagnosed with ADHD when she was young and finds life easier now she has access to medication.

I was diagnosed with ADHD as a child. But my parents – due to the stigma and total lack of support at the time – kept it hidden from me. Instead, they got me to channel all of my focus and energy into playing sports. Looking back, they were just doing what they thought was right at the time. When I was 'naughty' in school and couldn't sit still they would just call my mum and basically blame her for not 'controlling' me enough.

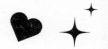

When I reached my late teens I began to recognise myself in ADHD stories. I told my parents and they admitted that, yes, I did have ADHD. But it had been so long since my diagnosis that I had to go through the process all over again. It was long, it took around six months and it cost about 700 euros. Paying for a private diagnosis is really the only option in Ireland. It's either that or languishing on a waiting list for years. After my diagnosis I went on medication, but it really didn't agree with me – it made me so anxious. I couldn't eat, had a constant headache, was losing so much weight. I thought, 'This is horrible,' and I quickly came off it and began to self-medicate instead with alcohol. I also stopped doing sports. I began to spiral. Eventually I was admitted to hospital with depression and my doctors dismissed all my problems as addiction issues. No one really brought up the ADHD.

Eventually I got a better psychiatrist. Together we began to experiment with my medication dosage until we found one that worked for me. Since taking it, while life is still hard at times, it's much more manageable. I'm no longer playing team sports, but I still like to keep active. I've got a job I love and a brilliant support system.

The Validity of Self-diagnosis

Between us we have clinical diagnoses, diagnoses that have come from therapists, and realisations following years of research and struggle that haven't ended in pursuing a clinical diagnosis. Let us say this: we think all are equally valid.

As we've talked about, getting an ADHD or autism diagnosis is HARD. The process is difficult for neurodivergent brains to manage, and the waiting lists are long. Even if you begin this process, even if your GP sends you the forms, you might not reach the end of the road. You might decide that, hell, your mental health (if it starts costing you that) is worth more than an 'official' diagnosis.

It's also worth knowing that there are some real-world consequences of having a diagnosis. While it's not a particularly nice thing to talk about, it feels as though we'd be doing you a disservice by not discussing some of the less great things that diagnosed autistics especially have to face. Ableism lives not only in the way society treats neurodivergent people interpersonally; it is also systemic. Some countries (like New Zealand, for example) restrict immigration access if people have disabilities that they deem a potentially high burden on the healthcare system, and autism is included in these criteria.[6] It was also the case that, during the COVID pandemic, thousands of Brits with learning disabilities were given a 'Do Not Resuscitate' status without their consent.[7] It goes without saying that these limitations and ableist policies don't affect every person with a medical diagnosis, but it's a reality for SOME autistics, and we feel like you deserve to be given the heads-up that you do need to research what that looks like before you make the decision to push forwards with a medical diagnosis.

If you do decide to go ahead with pursuing a medical diagnosis, you might choose to seek one through private healthcare (though not everyone can afford that) or via one of the charities that offer a diagnosis pathway, such as Psychiatry UK (although the list of those that do is ever-changing). In addition, many marginalised and oppressed communities might have previously felt dismissed by traditional healthcare systems and therefore might not feel comfortable using those same systems to pursue a diagnosis. This is why – regardless of your diagnostic status – we say that if you believe you have ADHD or autism, **WE BELIEVE YOU.** And we hope you believe us, too.

Diagnosis vs realisation

We put a lot of our trust in medical professionals, and often for good reason, but the difficulty lies in the fact that the medical system can be exclusionary of a lot of people. From our own experiences, as well as all the conversations we've had with people in our community, we can recognise how inaccessible getting a formal diagnosis can be for many people.

You'll often hear us refer to our ADHD and autism 'realisations' – we use this word as a way of putting the power back into our hands (and brain) to figure out for ourselves what works for us. Whether you can't pursue a diagnosis because you don't have access to a parent or someone who knew you during your childhood, or because the waiting list is already so long and you need help now, we understand that you will need to own your realisation and begin to craft your world to suit your needs without the help of a medical professional. Especially because we've heard of so many people – women and non-binary people especially – being fobbed off with 'Have you tried a planner?' and 'Here, try this leaflet' when they **do** reach the doctor's surgery. Why not realise how your brain works (or, as some call it, 'self-diagnose') and begin to figure out what you need for yourself?! If it's going to make you healthier and happier, go you.

Private healthcare has been touted as a 'solution' to the waiting-list problem, but many people, including us, don't have access to the money needed for a private diagnosis. If you have pursued one and got one, that's great, and we're delighted for anyone who does whatever works for them and follows their own path. For us, so much of this journey has been about going deeper than we've ever done before, and we did this through realisation and researching and educating ourselves, rather than formal advice and diagnosis from our doctors.

Jess on ... her autism realisation

When we first started I Am Paying Attention I was throwing myself into studying autism so that I could be a better advocate for Mia, who had already realised she was autistic after conversations with her therapist, and our community. But it was during some of these long chats with Mia that I began to realise that I could be autistic, too. So with a clinical ADHD diagnosis already under my belt, and the awareness that lots of information out there about being autistic wasn't inclusive of lots of us, I started trying to see if the shoe fitted when I read the work of autistics online.

Instead of reading this work and just considering it another part of wanting to be educated and better able to advocate for other people, I started processing it in a way that I hadn't before – and some really big fucking realisations came pouring in. There were parts of myself that **did** loosely fit with being stereotypically autistic, such as:

⚡ Being super sensitive to sounds that didn't bother anyone else for as long as I could remember.

⚡ Having huge amounts of knowledge in areas I'd been passionately interested in.

⚡ Having three predictable meals I'd eat over and over again for as long as I'd been cooking for myself.

⚡ Spotting patterns and almost being able to (correctly) foresee how certain situations would pan out, because I'd seen it before multiple times (I think this is why so many autistics are great digital strategists).

⚡ Collecting things, like train tickets, for 10-plus years.

⚡ Focusing on single projects for a long period of time, to the exclusion of others (called monotropism, see page 54).

I started realising that my hair-twirling habit was probably stimming (see page 55), and so was biting my lips and cuticles – and the way I rub my feet together when I'm trying to get comfy … Oh, and rubbing my thumbs against my fingertips. As I say, the revelations kept coming, and as they did I started to change my attitude towards these little self-regulating behaviours, celebrating them for the cute anxiety soothers or mood boosters they are.

I'm certain that I am autistic, but with the experience of getting a clinical ADHD diagnosis under my belt, I didn't feel like I could put myself through that again to get an autism diagnosis. The ADHD process had been utterly exhausting and it had required me to dig up some uncomfortable memories that I wasn't ready to process yet.

I'd seen others talk about their autism assessments, and many had found that those assessing them weren't up to date in their knowledge of what masked autism can look like. Because I'd already been on a journey of getting to know myself, I had the tools I needed to soothe myself without going through the medical diagnostic pathway. It's worth noting, though, that I work for myself, so I didn't 'need' a clinical diagnosis as proof to ask an employer for reasonable adjustments (see page 181), and if I did need to ask for adjustments at any point (e.g. in airports), I could do so on the grounds of my lupus and ADHD diagnoses.

As you can see, a lot of different and very personal factors played into my decision not to seek a formal diagnosis – and you might be on your own journey, mulling over some of these same aspects. I was leaning in to my needs more than I'd ever done before, and while life with responsibilities was still stressful, at least I now had tools to help me feel more **like me**, rather than the version of me that was always in a high state of stress. I also wanted to make sure I was showing others in our community that these things are not only natural, but also beautiful and fun.

Mia on ... her autism and ADHD realisations

As you'll have read on page 21, my self-diagnosis journey was rocky. It happened in a different way to Jess's, highlighting the differences in each person's route.

For a while, ignoring my own needs worked, but – as with all things you choose to ignore – eventually it bit me on the ass. When I started to suspect I had autism and ADHD, I began furiously researching every single aspect of it. Although I had the realisation very quickly, it took me quite a while to accept it. I spent so many months picking things apart that I actually ended up more confused than before.

I did try to pursue an ADHD diagnosis via the NHS, but I didn't have any support and found the process so inaccessible and detrimental to my mental health that I stopped. In the end, it was a therapist who suggested I was autistic and had ADHD. I'd been having some very deep and profound conversations with her and – given that there is no autism or ADHD blood test – I trusted her judgement, because it reflected my own feelings and I felt like I'd disclosed so much of my personal life to her that she was well placed to say.

My therapist gave me the only professional validation I've had on this journey, but in my eyes, she gave me the clarity and confirmation that I couldn't get from the systems that should have supported me.

As you can see, diagnoses and realisations come in many different forms and, while the research and healthcare infrastructure that we so desperately need is still catching up, we hope that this chapter has given you a sense of validation in your own experiences. Perhaps you'll decide that pursuing a clinical diagnosis is the right thing for you. Maybe you already have one and it's helped you. Or maybe you don't feel up to it right now or don't want to go down that road. Those choices are all entirely valid. Always remember: you do you.

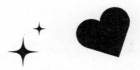

CHAPTER 6

To Mask or Not to Mask?

⚡ **What is masking?**

⚡ **Why mask?**

⚡ **The pros and cons of unmasking**

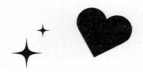

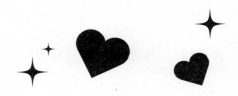

We were once chatting to a wonderful friend of ours, Lor, and explaining that we 'read other people's body language and then figure out exactly how we should respond'. She gently and kindly pointed out that treating communication like a maths equation was not our natural way of thinking and chatting. Instead, it must have been something we'd been studying for years. We just kind of figured that everyone was obsessed with reading psychology articles to learn how to be THE BEST, MOST SOCIABLE, CHATTIEST PERSON EVER. This is masking: or hiding or disguising parts of yourself in order to better fit in with those around you, according to the National Autistic Society.

Masking (and then unmasking) is tricky to try to unpick. According to Dr Hannah Belcher, writing for the National Autistic Society about her own experience alongside her research, masking or camouflaging is a natural thing **all** humans do. It's a way to better fit in with your peers. But when it comes to neuro-divergent people, she writes, 'the strategy is much more ingrained and harmful to our wellbeing and health'.[1] This is because our social norms are different from those around us, so we spend our entire lives mimicking and hiding our true selves. It's because we're afraid we will be discriminated against for being ourselves. It's also important to note that while the term 'masking' comes from the autistic community, many with ADHD will also mask, particularly those who have had a late diagnosis.

What can masking look like?

- ⚡ Not processing emotions outwardly (i.e. not crying).
- ⚡ Forcing eye contact or looking elsewhere.
- ⚡ Mimicking others' personal interests.
- ⚡ Scripting conversations ahead of time.
- ⚡ Copying gestures.

Ableism - and Internalised Ableism

Ableism is – put plainly – favouring so-called non-disabled people. Internalised ableism is when disabled people experience these feelings about themselves, believing that their disability and how it presents are something to be ashamed of or to hide. For example, you might have internalised messages you've received from society that because you can't work in neurotypical settings, it must mean you're 'lazy' or 'incapable'. It might be said that we mask as a result of our internalised ableism, because we don't feel our true disabled selves will be accepted and feel some shame about how our traits show up when we don't mask. Unlearning this internalised ableism – which might involve unmasking (see page 114) – is one of the kindest, most radical and transformative things you can do for yourself.

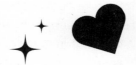

Our Major Masks (and How We Stopped Using Them)

Masking is often not a conscious choice, or something we proactively decide to do at all. If throughout your school years you've been asked to 'Stop fidgeting!' or 'Stop rocking on your chair?!' or been told, 'Look at me when I'm talking to you?!' then you might have internalised the idea that the things that come naturally to you – like fidgeting, or avoiding glaring deep into someone's shiny eyeballs mid-conversation – aren't what you're supposed to be doing.

While there are plenty of autistics who can't make eye contact at all, there are lots of us who have forced ourselves to do it, just trying to do as we're told and avoid getting ourselves into shit. A huge factor behind why both of us doubted that we were autistic for way too long was because we both thought we were incredible at communication. When we think about it now it's actually laughable, because what we really meant was that chatting between the two of us was easy. With everyone else, we were masking.

Jess

My major mask is people-pleasing! I'd centre everything on the other person, ensuring that they were happy and never once considering how I felt. Part of my unmasking journey has been realising that I don't need to be the unpaid therapist in my relationships. I don't need to give my energy and time to people who don't give back. This has meant that I've drifted from people, but the energy and freedom I feel from letting go of those relationships has been exceptional.

Mia

I really struggle with communication. Before, I'd just totally ignore my messages and pretend they weren't there, which led to my family and friends worrying about me. Now I have the right language to use – I know it's okay to reply and say, 'I can't really pinpoint how I'm feeling right now,' or even, 'My brain feels a little grey right now,' and my partner absolutely knows what I mean.

Mia on ... masking

Remember my weird 'rock' analogy from our introduction (see page 21)? Well, I'm now going to talk about the rock bottom I couldn't bring myself to process when writing Part 1.

I'll be honest, I went backwards and forwards on whether I even wanted to share this part of my life – because now it's just **out there** in the world for you to read. However, I know that if I've experienced this, then there's probably a shit load of you who have **also** experienced it, and if it gives anyone just a glimmer of hope then I'm happy.

In 2018 I relocated to Brighton and managed to hold down a job (for longer than a year!). I was paying rent and in a relationship. I was making friends. I thought each of these things was, at some point, the solution to my inability to feel consistently happy.

Then, over a series of months, each one of these things broke down. I still can't really piece together which came first, but I remember friendships feeling harder to maintain, which hurt because **most** of the friends I made were lovely. I also inevitably started slipping in my job. It started out as a manageable role that was still challenging enough for me to enjoy, but I gradually started sliding into a reality where I was burning out more quickly than I could complete any work.

I still go backwards and forwards thinking about the horrible idea that maybe if I had known then that I was autistic and ADHD, somehow I could have managed better. Then again, would I have even been hired if my boss had known I was ADHD and autistic? Probably not. I had many warnings and offers of support from teachers and managers over the years, but when it got down to it, I was essentially unable to function because I didn't know how I worked, so how was I ever going to be able to communicate that to anyone else?

At the same time, my mum's health was in a bad place, and as much as she told me over and over **and over** again that she was 'still my mum' and still there for me, it was difficult to navigate how honest I could be about how much I was struggling because of the stress I knew it would cause her.

Due to my inability to communicate with my family at the time, relationships got very strained; I've always been close to my mum – she's always been my number-one support – but during this period, it felt hard, and as though it wasn't going to get better.

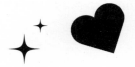

So, to summarise: I ended up losing contact with my friends, I lost my job, my relationship ended and my relationship with my family was extremely difficult. Oh, and I was behind on my rent, yippee! That, my friends, is a major fallout. And it all happened because at the time I was unaware of why I was struggling so much to maintain any sort of normality. I just kept going and ending up in the same cycles I mentioned earlier (and you can only do that so many times until you reach a point of pure exhaustion).

During this time, there was one question that chased me: 'But you used to be able to manage – why can't you anymore?' **Because I had been masking, that's why.** I was deeply clued up on what's needed to survive in this world; I've always been pretty good at reaching a point of perceived 'success'. I can work extremely hard to maintain a facade of normality. I can get jobs, make friends, forge relationships. But the effort and masking involved in actually keeping up that act is exhausting. So the real answer to that question is: 'It always looked like I was managing before, but I wasn't. I was masking!'

Unmasking

Okay, so you've realised that a lot of your behaviours – the shit you thought was natural and that **everyone** did – is masking. Now what? Unmasking can be an incredibly powerful thing to do. Remember what we said about studying people constantly, and working out the best way to respond? That's really fucking tiring. It's like we're computers with 20 other programs whirring away in the background. Eventually

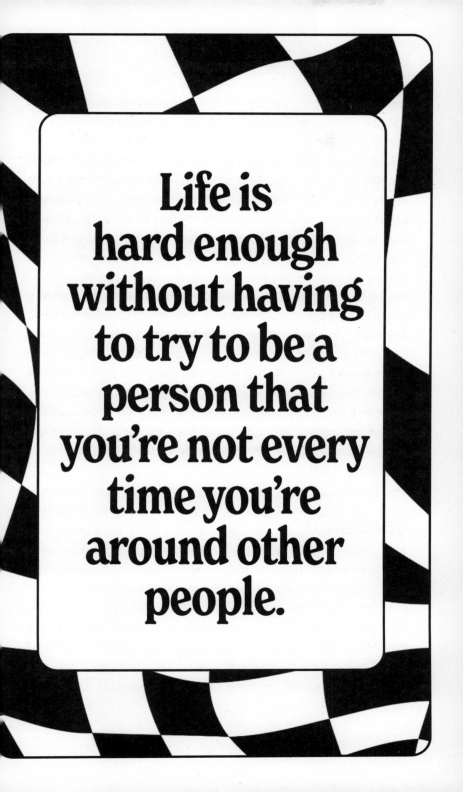

Life is hard enough without having to try to be a person that you're not every time you're around other people.

we're going to break down. Our operating systems can't handle that much!

But it's really not as simple as tearing off a mask and saying, 'Ta-da! This is the real me!' It's partly a huge victory that you know now that you've been masking, but it's also very complicated when you consider that, moving forwards, being authentic now looks very different. Once you realise that you work in a way you've actively been suppressing, it's likely that the only way you've got there is because you've had to dig **really** deep inside your brain to figure out what feels authentic and organic. Once that's clicked for you, you **might** also realise how rough life has been while you were suppressing things.

On the one hand, it kind of feels a bit like learning to walk from scratch, you know? On the other, it's liberating to realise that you can turn off the overhead lighting, reduce the noise and go from feeling like you're on the verge of ripping your hair out to actually noticing your shoulders drop.

You might start wearing sunglasses religiously every time you leave the house – because significantly reducing the brightness also seems to significantly reduce the 'I don't want to be here' thoughts. Maybe flicking a fidget toy through your hands while you get through those focus-heavy tasks actually makes them seem doable for the first time since … well … ever.

You could realise that your happy little excited hands, or your 'this food tastes so good I can't possibly contain it' dance, is actually a part of you that you should be able to enjoy – because, unless you're a child, **nothing** about it is childish.

You might realise that asking the people around you to reduce the multiple streams of noise (or putting in noise-cancelling headphones if you're able to get a hold of some) makes the world go from 100,000 on the overwhelming scale to at **least** half that.

So even if people around you don't understand or respect this journey the way you'd like them to, know that there are options – like leaving the damn room if they don't want to help you out. All of this might mean you finally get some respite from things that have been making life harder for you up until this point.

Why unmask?

If you're people pleasers like us, you may be wondering, 'Why unmask at all? People **like** me. I'm doing fine.'

Perhaps masking has got you far in life – it's got you a job, friends, relationships. But just because masking has been a reliable coping mechanism, that doesn't mean it's serving you. Not only have studies shown that autistic people who mask may be more prone to depression and anxiety,[2] but the strategy has even been linked to suicidal behaviours.[3] It's exhausting pretending to be someone you're not. It's also hiding who you really are from both yourself and others around you.

By unmasking, you'll get to know yourself better. We'll properly share in the rest of Part 2 what we've learnt about ourselves, and about where we should put our energy by unmasking, but we can tell you now: it's been truly freeing.

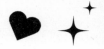

The dangers of unmasking

The thing is, while masking can come as such a relief, it's not possible for everyone all the time. As we've mentioned before (are you bored of us yet?!), we mask because it's what society expects of us. Behaving in our natural way could be perceived as odd or rude by others. And when you pair that with the other bullshit minority folks have to deal with on a daily basis, it could result in someone ending up in a dangerous situation. Remember the brilliant Morénike Giwa Onaiwu from Chapter 4, and those men who were attacked by the police (see page 71)? Those people were unmasking and it was seen as dangerous behaviour, and because America's gun laws are fucked up (to say the least) it got them killed. Young Black males are nearly three times more likely to be killed by police than their white counterparts.[4] And those who are autistic are seven times more likely to encounter the police than neurotypical individuals.[5] We once read a list of things that shoplifters do, which included observations like 'seems a little nervous' and 'picks up and puts down items' – these could also simply be soothing behaviours for someone who is neurodivergent.

So if someone is already targeted for their race and they're displaying these natural behaviours, they could end up attracting the radar of the security guard. Then there's the fact that, according to NHS data, Black people are four times more likely to be detained under the Mental Health Act than white people.[6] So be aware that being yourself and unmasking in public could lead you to display behaviours that some people perceive as wrong and hold against you. It's deeply distressing and unfair, and many more conversations about this need to be had.

Harri's Story

Harri, 32, from Liverpool, was formally diagnosed as autistic in February 2022 and discusses her experience of masking here.

I was seeking a diagnosis for PTSD (post-traumatic stress disorder) when it was floated to me that I could perhaps be autistic. At first, I was like, 'What?' But then the more I read, and certainly the more I read about how it presents in women and girls, I did begin to accept that perhaps my psychiatrist had been right. Things began to make a lot more sense in terms of my childhood and the way I viewed the world.

I didn't do anything with the knowledge for a while – but as I'm also currently studying, I thought if I had a formal diagnosis, I would be able to ask for what I need more. At that point, I'd come to a place of self-diagnosis and that was really helping me to make sense of my life. I kept thinking, 'What if they say I'm not?' I didn't want it taken away from me. One of my fears was definitely, 'They won't believe me when I talk about how I experience certain things.' I had a little bit of money at the time, so I decided to go private – and I had *such* a positive experience. Every step of the way it felt like the professionals I met were coming from a place where they believed me. That was so validating. But it's frustrating I had to spend so much money to get there.

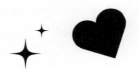

I'm a quiet person who doesn't want to take up too much space. I'm still getting to know the different ways that I mask. There are definitely many things I still do with people that I know I wouldn't do if I felt completely comfortable. My accent even changes sometimes. I'll rehearse conversations in my head before I have them, which is an extra layer to communication. But now it almost feels automatic to do that.

As a child I'd go to all of the birthday parties, even though I absolutely hated them, because I was expected to go. I'd want to be in the corner, or at home with my book, but I'd push myself into spaces and situations where I didn't feel safe or comfortable. I still do that a lot now, but, since my diagnosis, I have more awareness of it. I'll make decisions knowing my energy is going to be drained and work in time to relax afterwards.

One of the major reasons I mask is because I don't feel safe otherwise. It's a fear of rejection and highlighting that I don't really fit in. In my college there's fluorescent strip lights, and they really bother me and I want to wear sunglasses, but I just pretend it's okay, as putting on sunglasses would really shine a spotlight on me. There are so many expectations placed on us as women – particularly non-white women like me. If we don't behave in a certain way, we're labelled rude, angry or difficult. It's so scary to open yourself up to that sort of criticism.

I sometimes think, 'Oh, maybe I don't give people enough credit,' that maybe others would get it and understand. But also, I'm not sure I want to be the sort of person to have to educate others. I have a huge respect for Jess and Mia as they're showing up and exploring their journeys in a public space, but that's a huge responsibility. I often feel I only have my personal experience, with not a lot of research or data to back it up. All I can say is: 'This is what it feels like to be me.' That should be enough for people, but I'm worried about putting myself into situations where it's maybe not.

It's scary to think of the real-life consequences unmasking could have if I come across anyone with outdated and untrue notions of what autism is.

The Long-lasting Impact

Long-term masking puts us in a state of constant stress – how can we be expected to be relaxed when we're pretending to be someone we're not? Now we are being our authentic selves life feels calmer somehow. Like many other ND people, we've also experienced confusion over which parts of ourselves are masking and which are truly us, because masking has become such a big part of who we are. This has a dissociative effect, where we struggle to connect our thoughts and feelings into one coherent life story. Not knowing what is your 'real' personality and what isn't can be very dehumanising.

We get it. You could easily look at us from the outside, through the 'display' window of Instagram, and think, 'Yeh, they've really got it together.' Our IG is curated. We post pictures of ourselves in fun outfits. We got a goddamn book deal! Even when we're being vulnerable on Instagram, those posts are still neatly presented and articulated with intention. But that image projection doesn't match up with the reality. Because even now that we know we have autism and ADHD, we still fall into masking behaviours all the time. As we've talked about, masking sometimes functions to keep us safe in a society that isn't always accommodating for neurodiverse people. Knowing you're autistic or ADHD doesn't always prompt an unmasking celebration – it's far more nuanced than that. Even though you know the source of your exhaustion, there's a realisation that this isn't something you can 'fix' and this point is often where the judgement really begins.

Whether or not you choose to continue masking, to unmask fully or to be a little selective and unmask slowly over time is a totally personal choice, but we hope that we've given you a flavour of what to expect, whichever route you take. As always, do what serves YOU best – it's your journey, and nobody else's.

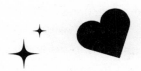

CHAPTER 7

Grief and Burnout

⚡ **The grieving process**

⚡ **Recognising neurodivergent burnout**

⚡ **Dealing with burnout**

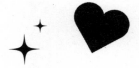

If we had to sum up our grief in one sentence, it would be this: **Maybe if I'd known I was neurodivergent, I wouldn't have carried pain like this for so long.**

Much like a big regret or losing someone close to you, finding out something later on in life that has altered the path of your very existence can be distressing.

After all, you're sorting through the what-ifs and navigating the fact that something crucial to your knowledge and understanding of who you are and how you experience the world has been missed. We've had quite a few conversations about grief during our healing process. Grieving for our past selves, and the versions of us that didn't have the confidence we have now – the versions who'd stay quiet when they didn't understand. We've spent time thinking about the opportunities those people didn't get and where we might be now if that hadn't been the case. Or where the relationships that failed might've ended up if we'd known how to navigate life with this understanding. The shit that many of us have to grapple with leaves us with less money, less security and, often, a string of bad relationships that have chipped away a huge chunk of our confidence. We're grieving those losses as well.

Internalised Ableism and Grief

A huge part of accepting an ADHD and autism realisation or diagnosis is being able to admit that there are some things you'll struggle to manage – such as making plans with friends or keeping up with life admin. And that no matter how many techniques or time-management apps you use, no matter how hard you fucking try, there are parts of society that will not accept you.

Your internalised ableism plays into this because, for a long time, you will have wanted to change. You'll have seen not being able to do these things as a failure on your part. Understanding the ableism in the standards we were holding ourselves to was crucial to our healing. If we were **still** holding ourselves to those standards, we wouldn't be able to do the work we do. We know lots of people who are post-realisation or diagnosis who still struggle with their own internalised ableism and their desire to adhere to neurotypical standards, and it blights their lives and their ability to carve out what they need. But once you realise the role that internalised ableism plays and accept that a realisation or diagnosis of ADHD or autism will probably mean that you become less productive, less 'useful' to society, because you're not working yourself to the point of burnout, it makes grieving your circumstances easier.

This is a really hard thing to come to terms with. You may find yourself fighting it, masking the grittier parts of your reality. Particularly if you have friends and family around you who also have internalised ableism, who try 'helpfully' to suggest that 'perhaps if you just tried [insert really obvious bullshit sugges-tion here]' then everything would be different. It's taxing and makes the whole process of getting to grips with your grief so much harder.

Our Five Stages of Grief

You might have heard of the five stages of grief, a model created in the 1960s by psychiatrist Elisabeth Kübler-Ross, which states that we **all** go through five different stages of grief.[1] While often cited relating to bereavement, the five stages were actually formed when discussing what people go through when it comes to the dying process. It's also been criticised in the past as adding unnecessary pressure for us to grieve in the 'right' way, when, of course, there's no right or wrong way to process our own emotions. Listing them as consecutive stages also confused people – what if they jumped straight to one, and missed out another? What if they went through one, only to circle back round to it a few months later? So, when reading through our own stages of grief that follow, know this: we don't all go through them in the same order and they can often repeat themselves. And other things can also come into play that often cloud the judgement throughout this process.

Shock and denial

For those who haven't been searching for an ADHD or autism diagnosis, shock may be the first emotion they feel when they find out, but, for many of us, researching labels like ADHD and autism comes before we're diagnosed by a professional or realise it for ourselves. It goes without saying that this isn't always the case, but for those of us who go looking for an answer, shock isn't always the first thing we feel.

Denial, for us, meant we invalidated our own feelings. Even after hours and hours of research (not to mention launching a whole community surrounding our ADHD and autism!), we could find ourselves asking internal questions such as, 'But am I really autistic or just lying to myself?!' This is actually quite understandable when we think about how we'd never really seen neurodivergence look like **us** before. Remember: just because it isn't represented doesn't mean it doesn't exist.

Pain and guilt

Once you understand the truth behind your past (or others' past) behaviours, you'll find a lot of pain resurfaces. Like a lot of people, we'd been in a state of high alert – fight-or-flight mode – for a really long time, and once we had our realisations it felt like the first time we'd really been able to press pause, sit with it all and gain some perspective.

You might be feeling for the younger version of you who wasn't given the respect or access to things they deserved, and it's an entirely reasonable thing for you to feel hurt over that mistreatment – especially if you've started thinking about what could've been. You might, like us, reflect on relationships and realise that although you were doing your best with what you had, you've actually been the one causing pain – and that's a bit of a tough pill to swallow, too.

Or maybe you're looking at people **you** resented and seeing them in a different light. Needless to say, this phase came with a lot of regret and some really rough insights for us.

Anger

To get past the pain and the guilt we were hefting around with us, we looked at situations with a different, lighter perspective – one that finally took the blame off our shoulders. Sounds great, right? Well, actually, it wasn't. It had us pretty seething over what had gone on, and how we'd been made to feel by others. It wasn't always rational, but we can only say that now because ... **healing**.

We felt misdirected anger – anger at the rest of society for making us feel as though neurotypical standards were ones we should be able to meet, anger at the people who **were** able to manage life under those conditions and, honestly, sometimes even at those close to us for not understanding things the way we did (even though it was **our** journey).

There were plenty of heightened emotions going on when we were at this stage. We can admit now that this meant we had less capacity to empathise with others, particularly when it came to recognising that there were people around us who didn't have first-hand, lived experience of all the new pieces of information we had immersed ourselves in. This meant that they didn't understand us as clearly as we needed them to ... and that was frustrating at times.

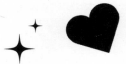

We'd regularly be exhausted by the internal work we were doing, and so often we noticed resentment building when we found ourselves having to educate other people – because it's one thing unlearning your ableist preconceptions about how things should be, and relearning what is actually right for you, but feeling like you have to justify your existence to others, especially to people you care about, is another entirely.

Depression

It's no secret that being neurodivergent often seems to come with a package deal of various mental illnesses – at least at some point in our lives, anyway. Plenty of us floated around for years feeling depressed or anxious (or both), questioning why the fuck we couldn't chill out or even if things were ever going to get better.

Upon learning this new information about how our brains worked, we felt some relief. But that relief wasn't a cure – it didn't suddenly take away all the difficult things that come with being disabled. In fact, studies have found that you're more likely to have depression if you are disabled.[2]

On the one hand, it was fascinating and comforting when we started to have conversations with people who understood, or were at a similar place in their journey – however, there were also people in our lives who mean a lot to us but who **weren't** where we were at, and feeling misunderstood by those you love can hugely trigger low mood and poor mental health, too. That shit is difficult to navigate – probably on both sides.

We've also had plenty of conversations with each other where we've had to pull ourselves out of the Big Bad Depression Hole after we've realised that it's actually an extremely grim reality to be disabled in a world like this one, and no matter how positive we are, that reality won't change overnight.

The upward turn

By this stage, the anger and pain have often died down, and you're left in a calmer and more relaxed state.

What happens if you circle back?

Sorry to break it to you, but you might. Grief doesn't work like a checklist where you go through, say, anger and then you get to scratch it off your list. But what we can tell you is that each and every time you circle back, you're **not** back in the exact same place as before. You'll have learnt coping mechanisms from the last time you were in that space; even the fact that you're recognising your emotions is a huge step forward. It's also perfectly okay to feel pissed off, sad, emotional – you don't need to feel okay **all** the time to be moving forward. And remember, you don't need to struggle to be autistic or have ADHD. Sometimes we're so used to our experiences being difficult that we doubt ourselves when we're feeling at peace, but you're just as neurodivergent when you're not struggling as when you are.

Understanding your brain for the first time in your life, and knowing how to use it to approach everyday things so they no longer feel like a massive uphill struggle, is a very powerful feeling.

Jess on ... grief

I had already gone through one health grieving process: when I was diagnosed with the autoimmune condition lupus, during my university years. I had already let go of the idea that I could ever live a 'normal' life where I didn't have to think constantly about what I was eating or doing to my body. So there are days now when I think I'm totally at peace. When I don't feel I'm grieving for the life that could have been. I've reached a point where I know my struggles are society's problem, not mine. I used to resent that a lot, but now I've accepted it.

Mia on ... grief

I have days when I feel I'm no longer grieving, but then a life event will happen and catapult me backwards. It's very similar to how you grieve a person – there are moments in life that will remind you of your grief and fling you back into that space. When I look at the grief stages all mapped out I know I've gone through all of them, but I now know that the grieving process doesn't ever end – that there are elements of our lives that we have processed and healed, and if we do end up feeling bad again, we'll know we can get through them.

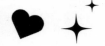

Burnout

If you're a human being, the chances are you've **probably** experienced burnout to some degree, at least once in your life.

However, experiencing prolonged periods of burnout, over and over again, was one of the signs that made us both realise something was **off**, because life really didn't seem to be THIS exhausting for the majority of people around us.

We'd find ourselves feeling like we were doing life on an expert level but as an absolute amateur. We'd have no motivation for long periods of time, and we'd always try to rationalise away how we were feeling. We'd tell ourselves we were burnt out because:

- ⚡ We'd been working late each night.
- ⚡ We'd poured all our energy into our relationships, leaving no time for anything else.
- ⚡ We were struggling with money.

And the confusing thing is, **all** of those reasons were true. But there was also, of course, the underlying reason. The thing we weren't yet aware of: that our autism and ADHD made life so much more taxing for the pair of us.

Neurodivergent burnout

A lot of us don't tend to pursue a diagnosis for ADHD or autism until we reach a point of breakdown or burnout – and neurodivergent burnout is a different breed altogether (see the list below for some tell-tale signs). Being overly emotional and irritable, but also numb and finding it so hard to verbalise those feelings, means it can be really hard to reach out and ask for help.

What Does Autistic Burnout Look Like?

We asked our community, and this is what they had to say about what burnout looks like for them. It's so validating having these conversations, as we know we're not alone in our experiences.

- ⚡ Not being able to meet my basic needs of hygiene, nutrition, social contact.
- ⚡ Knowing you have a deadline to meet and being highly anxious about it.
- ⚡ Overwhelming reams of thoughts and worries.
- ⚡ Not being able to get out of bed, even to eat.
- ⚡ Meltdowns over the smallest thing.
- ⚡ Being too tired to speak or even text.
- ⚡ Total anxiety when a loved one is calling.
- ⚡ Safe-food binge-eating.
- ⚡ A sense of being frozen and not able to start a task.
- ⚡ Can't figure out what I'm feeling! Like my head will explode if I don't scream or cry.
- ⚡ Sugar cravings.
- ⚡ Having no motivation for long periods of time.
- ⚡ Neglecting needs for a prolonged period (a common result of monotropic behaviours – see page 54).

There's no doubt that people with ADHD experience burnout and we know people in our community who have been through it, but in this section we're focusing specifically on autistic burnout because what research there is (and, you guessed it, there isn't much) gives a clearer picture on why and how autistic people specifically experience burnout. However, if you have ADHD or think you might and you're going through burnout, you deserve support and understanding. If you could benefit from the help that is available to you, take it – without shame. We hope that the advice in this section gives you some guidance.

There's been little research into what causes autistic burnout and how to combat it (surprise, surprise ...), but in a study published in the journal **Autism**,[3] an Australian research team led by Samuel Arnold from the University of New South Wales dug into it a little more. Here's what they discovered ...

- ⚡ **The most common burnout experience is withdrawal:** The survey spoke to 141 participants with a formal autism diagnosis (64 per cent female, 16 per cent male and 20 per cent reporting another gender) and asked them a range of questions about how much they related to autistic burnout. The most highly endorsed items relating to the burnout experience were to do with social withdrawal; for example, 'I felt extremely tired,' or 'I withdrew from social situations.'
- ⚡ **Our environment plays a huge part:** The things that the study found most contributed to autistic burnout? Stress ... and sensory environment challenges, with statementsincluding 'being overloaded by sensory and social information in my environment'. We hard relate.

⚡ **Burnout is physical:** As well as presenting specific examples, the survey also asked people to write their own comments and discovered a common thread within them. People described their burnout in a physical way, with light-headedness and dizzy spells being incredibly common. They also said they often found it really difficult to know when burnout was coming.

⚡ **Downtime is essential:** That feeling of needing to withdraw from social situations? It's probably a warning sign from your body. As the study found, participants said taking downtime and saying no to social stuff was their best coping mechanism.

Ways to avoid burnout

One of the toughest things when it comes to burnout and recovering from it is how much privilege comes into play, as one of the main ways to recover is to let your nervous system rest by taking time off. This isn't possible for everyone for a myriad of reasons, from childcare issues to needing to pay the rent. That's why some people remain in a state of burnout for years and years.

While some people think burnout is just feeling tired because you have a lot on at work, in reality it's ignoring your basic needs for a prolonged period of time. One technique Mia learnt is to write down in her planner her basic needs – showering, eating three meals a day – to try to make sure she meets them.

How to Get Through Neurodivergent Burnout

Some techniques recommended by the National Autistic Society include:

⚡ **Using energy accounting:** This is about looking, realistically, at how much energy you have in a week and what you're going to use it on, and working out what activities drain you and what ones give you energy. It's a gradual process to figure all that out, but once you have you can set a limit on what you can do that week. And learn that most vital word: no.

⚡ **Keeping track of your workload:** Jot down the hours you're working, and the tasks you're doing. This can then be used as a way to chat to your manager (if it's work that's overwhelming you to the point of burnout) and figure out a way to manage their expectations.

⚡ **Unmasking time:** Suppressing behaviours like stimming is exhausting, but there are some situations where you may feel like you have to do them. So ensure you also put in rest time that allows you to be your whole self.

Pauline Harley, the career coach and support group leader we met in Chapter 3, suffered with chronic burnout for decades before realising it was autistic burnout when she was diagnosed at 45. 'Burnout can happen for a number of reasons, from feeling the need to mask and adopt different personalities in the workplace, to becoming so hyperfocused on the task that you cannot recognise when you need breaks,' she says. 'There's also the sensory environments, and social hangovers, and it can also happen when you're really passionate about something and want to work to your limit on that.' Luckily, says Pauline, it is possible to get out of it by managing the expectations of others (and those you put on yourself), reframing your time and becoming more compassionate about how some things may take you longer. 'Think, how can I advocate for my needs in a way that's within my control and reasonable?' she says.

Three things to remind yourself of if you are feeling burnt out

The thing we really want to emphasise here is how important it is to be softer with yourself. If you end up in a state of burnout, it's not your fault.

- ⚡ You are a human being, not a machine. You're allowed to have fluctuating energy levels.
- ⚡ As neurodivergent people, we often have trouble noticing our body's cues (more on this in Chapter 13), which can make it pretty easy to miss the signs that we need to rest! Take baby steps towards discovering what tired looks like for you.
- ⚡ You are, in fact, worth more than the comfort you provide for other people. Save some energy for yourself.

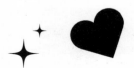

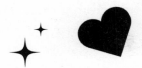

CHAPTER 8

Dealing with the Fallout

⚡ **Processing trauma**

⚡ **Coping mechanisms**

⚡ **Finding your safe people**

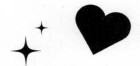

The truth is that, prior to our realisation or diagnosis, we often attributed many of the difficulties we faced to personal failings, and that's a heavy load to carry. As much as there's a feeling of relief that you now have **an answer** (sort of), there are also lots of tricky emotions that come attached to it. It came as a bit of a shock to us that we had to pour so much energy into processing ALL of them. That's what we mean by the fallout – all the stuff you have to work through, post-realisation or diagnosis, which involves retracing your steps and re-examining your history, as well as looking forward to what your future might be.

We're going to try to fill you in on all we've learnt while dealing with our own personal fallouts, as well as harness the advice of others we've met along the way. But first, of course, we want to check our privilege, as we know that, in some ways, we have been fortunate in our experiences, and that has meant that our fallouts have been easier than they might have been.

Our privileges include:

- ⚡ Being self-employed, which is kind of because we kept being fired, but we digress – it gives us a freedom we know some might not have.
- ⚡ Being white.
- ⚡ Being cisgender (we identify as the sex we were assigned at birth).

- ⚡ Having partners with their own income.
- ⚡ Having access to a solid emotional support
  network.

These things mean that we're in a better position to cope with the fallouts of ADHD and autism than many others, but trust us when we tell you that living in a world that isn't built for neuro-divergent people is still far from easy; it's often painful, and completely and utterly debilitating to navigate. It often leaves us unable to:

- ⚡ speak
- ⚡ work
- ⚡ wash regularly
- ⚡ eat without being prompted or cooked for
- ⚡ regulate our feelings
- ⚡ keep hold of any energy to proactively enjoy our personal
  lives

All of which are useful things to be able to manage, really.

The same is true for so many of us in this community – and while our recent working environments have allowed us to be much more honest about our needs, we're still living in a world that **point blank** refuses to acknowledge that some of us simply move more slowly, particularly in the workplace.

There are certain expectations of us that are so deeply embed-ded in our society that they show up regularly in our work, schools, universities and personal lives. And when even the most well-intentioned person can hurt us without even realising they're doing it, well ... it can sometimes feel like you're wading through a lot of shit.

All of that said, there are some factors that might make the fallout harder for you. They're the same factors that might mean you mask for longer (see Chapter 6):

- ⚡ **Caring for people:** If you're someone who has people who depend on you to care for them, your capacity to work through trauma is probably going to be significantly less.
- ⚡ **Your career and financial position:** If you are someone who works three jobs in an attempt to pay the bills, it might feel like there's no room left for you to worry about how your brain works. Whether we like it or not, we live in a society that equates productivity with worth, which means that if you're in a precarious financial position or are experiencing career instability, the fallout is likely to be worse.
- ⚡ **Your race and sexuality:** When you're already having to navigate racism or homophobia and then there's another layer of stress to consider, you may find it scary to unmask, as it means drawing attention to yourself.

Ultimately, the fallouts of realisation, getting a diagnosis, masking and unmasking look different for everyone, so ... Be! Kind! To! Yourself!

Just because you see someone else dealing with their fallout in a different way to you, that doesn't mean you're processing things badly or wrongly.

Trauma

We've mentioned trauma and feeling traumatised a few times so far, but how do trauma and neurodivergence actually intersect?

Psychologist and author of **How to Do the Work** Nicole LePera describes trauma as 'the result of a deeply catastrophic event'.[1] She says: 'The reality is that there are many people who cannot point to several moments (or even one moment) that broke their life apart. Many might not be able to admit that any part of their childhood was damaging. That doesn't mean that there wasn't trauma present – I've yet to meet a person who has not experienced some level of trauma in their life. I believe that our understanding of trauma should be widened to include a diverse range of overwhelming experiences.'

We've been friends for 10 years and talked about a lot during that time, but the idea that we've been dealing with trauma as well as our spicy neurodivergent brains didn't occur to us until quite recently – and that's probably because conversations about both things are thankfully becoming more normalised, and descriptions like LePera's one above have given us the language and the validation to understand that we are holding on to trauma.

When we first had our ADHD/autistic realisations, many painful things from the past suddenly made sense in a way we'd never anticipated: the way we often felt too much, or not enough; the way we couldn't manage what so many others around us could;

the consistent feelings of not being able to catch up and being completely exhausted most of the time as we tried. We unpacked these experiences through a neurodivergent lens. It was really affirming and validating, but it didn't dawn on us that all of the healing we'd been doing STILL wasn't addressing the full picture. **The more we've learnt about ourselves, the more we've realised that we're carrying trauma, too.**

Although we were aware that not all trauma looked the same, we had this idea that it would be more ... obvious. Surely if we had trauma, we'd know what it was, right? Actually, no. Learning about trauma through the work of people like LePera has made us realise that many of the things we'd struggled with **weren't** solely down to our neurodivergence but, as she says, being part of a marginalised group, which does make you more vulnerable to trauma because of how neurotypical societies treat us: 'When you live in a world that is unsupportive and outright threatening – in the education system, prison system, health care system, and most workplaces – you are existing in an almost constant state of trauma. Marginalised groups, especially BIPOC, are navigating systemic oppression, discriminatory laws, and a prejudicial framework that may place them squarely into a state of relative helplessness.' Although LePera rightly focuses on the experiences of ethnic minorities as victims of trauma, neurodivergent people like us have also been marginalised and live in an unsupportive society.

The research supports this: autistic people are more likely to report symptoms of PTSD and the rates of probable PTSD in autistic people (32–45 per cent) are higher than those in the general population (4–4.5 per cent).[2] According to the National

Autistic Society, 'Autistic people may be more likely to experience traumatic life events, particularly interpersonal traumas such as bullying and physical and sexual abuse,'[3] which leave us at increased risk of PTSD.

While some autism and ADHD traits are very definitely neurological differences, some of our experiences and traits have been enhanced by the trauma of neurotypical socialisation. For example, if you live in a family unit that invalidates your internal experiences, the likelihood that you're going to feel traumatised is going to be considerably higher. Some traits, such as rejection sensitive dysphoria (RSD) – an overwhelming fear of rejection – which for a long time has been considered a feature of ADHD, might also be a result of trauma, rather than an innate 'symptom' of ADHD brains. And as the statistics we've just mentioned indicate, living in a neurotypical society can have even more extreme and horrifying consequences.

These evolving conversations are still throwing up some questions that no one has the answers to: Do autistics and ADHDers who aren't traumatised exist? Are all humans traumatised to some extent? One thing we do know is that, as neurodivergent people, we are more vulnerable to feelings of trauma, so if this is resonating with you, go easy on yourself, know that it's not your fault, and seek support from kind and non-judgemental sources.

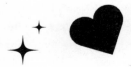

Shame

Shame is just one of the emotions you might be dealing with as part of the fallout from your ADHD/autism discovery, and it's a biggie. So let's take a deeper dive into how feelings of shame and having a neurodivergent brain can intersect.

This journey has many different aspects of shame attached to it – from not achieving the things you wanted to and having to process why, to dealing with the stigma still attached to things like medication or support. 'There is so much shame,' says career coach Pauline Harley. 'Shame of difference, shame of not fitting in, shame of being labelled "the difficult one".'

Unfortunately, there just isn't a recipe for managing shame, or an easy solution that we can deliciously roll into words to present to you, because the reality is that managing shame actually looks a lot like being okay with who you are, and we know you don't need us to tell you that shit isn't straightforward.

It looks like slowly understanding what you don't like about yourself, feeling your feelings and then processing them (rather than just analysing them). It also looks like shifting what you expect of yourself, even when other people are still expecting the same from you. 'Often we feel shame due to external expectations placed on us,' says Pauline. 'So it's about thinking to yourself, "I'm going to manage my expectations; they're mine, no one else's." It's about waking up each morning and saying, "I accept myself and my expectations in that space." Shame is usually from an external judgement and while it can be easy to

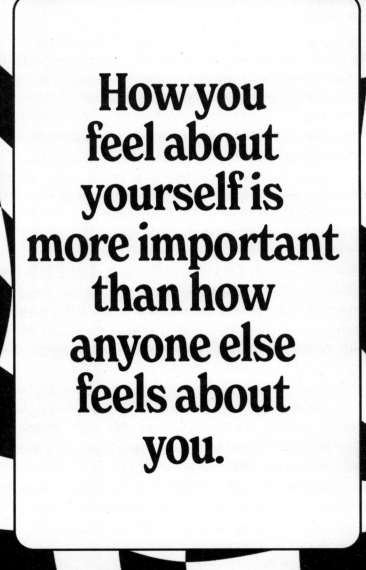

How you feel about yourself is more important than how anyone else feels about you.

think and judge the person making us feel that way, it's also important to own and recognise where we're letting shame in to our own detriment.'

It's a slow journey, but it's one that requires the gentleness and patience you were never able to give yourself before you had these insights. Honestly, in a world where we have access to so many other people's potentially shaming opinions and reflections at the tap of our silly little handheld computers, we're not sure it's a journey that ever ends.

We're always going to be able to compare ourselves to others, but maybe we can be a little quicker to interrupt any self-deprecating thoughts when we do with some affirming ones instead.

Managing shame is about overhauling your entire way of thinking; for example, reframing the thoughts you have in the shower from 'I'm such a piece of shit for not getting into the shower before 4 p.m.' to 'I really don't enjoy this task but I managed it – it took lots of little steps to get here and time is kind of a made-up, bullshit concept anyway, so I'll shower when I want'.

If all this isn't clear enough, completely reframing thoughts that have evolved over years of absorbing other people's shitty expectations **isn't** an easy task for our traumatised brains, so don't expect yourself to be able to manage it in a short period of time.

We've consistently reflected on whether, actually, it is quite understandable that we often find ourselves in a deeply over-whelming place when there are SO many demands placed upon us daily, such as:

- ⚡ Waking up at a certain time.
- ⚡ Feeding yourself adequate nutrition (and obtaining the ingredients to make it), also within a set timeframe.
- ⚡ Washing.
- ⚡ Cleaning our teeth.
- ⚡ Deciding what clothes to wear (and having clean ones, which also requires more labour).
- ⚡ Icky sensory shit like moisturising (oh, and you'd BETTER not forget your SPF or you're the devil incarnate).
- ⚡ Maybe even painting your face, because otherwise people might ask if you're okay or suffering from some other human 'flaw' like tiredness.
- ⚡ The mental gymnastics that come with trying to earn money in a job that doesn't make you miserable so you can survive.
- ⚡ The communication that comes with said job.
- ⚡ Maintaining relationships.
- ⚡ Hydrating.
- ⚡ Making your home look like nobody lives there 24/7.

Do you see our point? There's so much pressure in this world, it can feel like we're just endlessly checking things off of a never-ending to-do list, and, when we take a step back from that list, not a lot of what we're expected to do actually aligns up with what makes for a happy, healthy life. So if you're feeling overwhelmed try to remember that you, your health and your capacity for joy and love is what matters ... not the silly, trivial demands that we're told makes a 'good' life (but actually really don't).

Coping Mechanisms

After having regular conversations about the utter nonsense we've been tricked into having to do EVERY single day – and the fact that we're expected to still have energy left over to 'SMASH THAT SIDE HUSTLE' (sorry if we triggered you there ...) or 'MOVE YOUR BODY, NO EXCUSES!!!' – we've come to realise that while some people might possess brains that manage those demands a little more easily, it's completely exhausting for everyone, full stop.

That, my friends, is how we're managing shame. We no longer think we should be ashamed of struggling, because life is hard and it expects a lot from all of us.

Accepting that we want to move more slowly than is expected of us, and trying to make decisions that align with that **without** being sorry about it, has been incredibly healing in itself.

In the next part of this book, we'll be talking about how we navigate different areas of our lives – from the workplace to friendships – but here, we're going to spend a little bit of time discussing the general things that might make coping with the fallout that little bit easier.

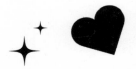

What we're saying no to (a never-ending list to be added to):

⚡ 'Advice' on various time-management strategies that bear no relation to our life right now.

⚡ The pressure to keep on top of domestic chores.

⚡ People in the fitness industry who are making money from people's fear of not being good enough – all while they loosely imply that we're just not trying hard enough so stop being a lazy piece of shit.

Don't get us wrong, we like a few practical tips too – just with less of the aggression and blame placed on our shoulders and more of the gentle 'Here's what we've figured out as exhausted humans – try it and see if it resonates.'

What we're saying yes to:

⚡ Accepting that we are doing 'enough' – and finally sitting with how reasonable it is that we're utterly exhausted.

⚡ Being gentle with ourselves and listening to our needs.

⚡ Sure, it's great if you can find ways to implement some habits that truly make your life feel better, but our personal experience tells us that comes with tuning in to our own individual requirements.

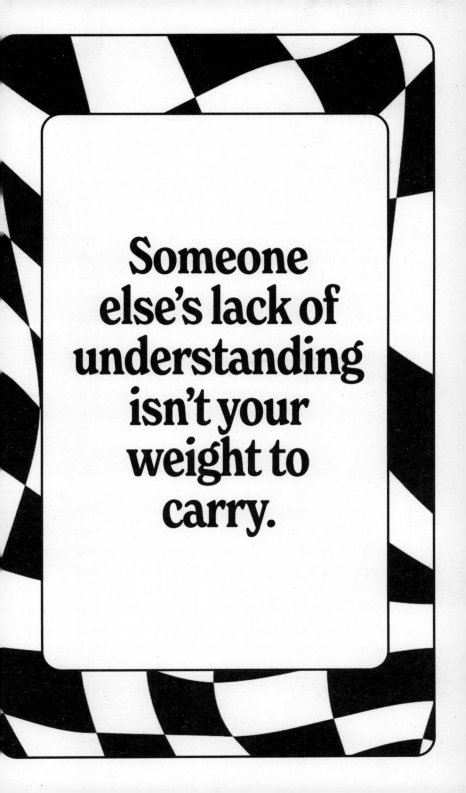

Someone else's lack of understanding isn't your weight to carry.

Finding Your Safe People

Sometimes, when we write about this topic, we worry that we're bringing you problems rather than solutions – and we know you don't need any more problems! The reality, however, is that we can't authentically bring you along with us to the place of (mostly) peace that we now experience without first acknowledging the painful parts, you know? Whether we like it or not, processing our struggles does hurt. The good news? We all have each other.

However your brain works, whether it's due to trauma, ADHD, autism, dyslexia, dyscalculia or dyspraxia, you deserve to get to know yourself and hold yourself to standards that **you** intentionally set for yourself. But once you've done that, finding your people, a community, can really help. And sometimes that community will help you get to know yourself even better than you could on your own. Wild, huh?

After all, we started I Am Paying Attention because we could not have gone through this journey without each other. The only way the painful parts hurt less was by shining some validation and perspective on what we'd experienced – and that's often hard to do alone, especially when you're already knee-deep in overwhelming feelings.

Western society seems to have this infatuation with hyper-independence, insisting that we are entirely fine without depending on anyone else. The problem with this is that so many of us DO need help – and we shouldn't have to battle feelings of inadequacy or inferiority every time we realise something is too difficult for us to manage alone. We're all too aware that what we're touching on here is a lot to digest, and very uncomfortable to work through, but we can wholeheartedly say this is a journey that has changed us and our lives in ways we could never have dreamed of.

Without wanting to sound too cheesy, when it comes to finding our safe people a huge part of our journey has involved finding ourselves first. Ensuring that we feel safe in our own company and know our own boundaries and needs (and feel utterly confident that they are right for us) makes it so much easier to communicate those needs to others. It also makes us better able to recognise the people in our lives who make us feel all cosy, fluffy and happy.

We'll get to how to navigate the situation when the people you love and care for carry stigma or ableism, and how to speak to them about that (turn to Chapter 11), but for now, know that safe people are out there and finding them will help. There are truly no words that'll ever come close to describing how comforting it is to feel like you finally have a home full of people who see you as **enough** exactly as you are.

The online community

So much of getting to where we are now has been thanks to the people we've met online. Without all the knowledge we now have about ADHD and autism, we couldn't have got to a place where we're able to embrace who we **actually** are, regardless of what box we fit into.

We've absorbed the words of so many autistic experts, researchers and those who run neurodivergent-focused Instagram accounts like ours. And while there's balance to be found when it comes to looking at your identity and pulling it apart (because, take it from us, it can make you feel more like a collection of labels than a **human being**), there's no disputing that finding your spot in a community of people you relate to can help you no end. In that safe, welcoming space you can give yourself grace, and learn about who you are, how you work and how you can tailor your life to make you feel more comfortable – both in your surroundings and with who you are. We've included a list of our favourite accounts to follow in the Resources section at the back of the book.

The Part 2 Workbook

What Happens Next?

Chapter 5: Do You Need a Diagnosis?

1. If you haven't got a medical diagnosis but you'd like one, do you have any worries, hang-ups or frustrations about the process? Example: Do you struggle with the admin involved?

   ....
   ....
   ....

2. If you have got a medical diagnosis, are you glad you made that decision? Did you expect life after diagnosis to be different? Example: What has changed since diagnosis for you? Has it changed anything for the better?

   ....
   ....
   ....

3. Considering your circumstances, can you think of any particular benefits to being medically diagnosed? (This isn't a trick question and 'no' is also a very valid answer!) Example: Have you been able to access the support you need?

....

....

....

Chapter 6: To Mask or Not to Mask?

1. Without stating the obvious, it definitely isn't always as straightforward as deciding to unmask and just ... doing it. Are there any particular spaces where you feel safe to do that? And equally, are there certain places you know it won't be safe for you to do so? And in those (shitty) circumstances, are there any ways you can subtly honour your needs without compromising your safety? Example: Perhaps you feel comfortable unmasking around your partner, but you may not feel safe to unmask in front of your family.

....

....

....

2. Is there anyone in particular you feel comfortable
   unmasking around? Why do you think that might be?
   Example: Similar to above, let's say it's your partner: Is
   that because they take time to listen? What do they do
   that your family don't?

   ....

   ....

   ....

3. Do you know when you're masking? It's all too easy for
   us to encourage unmasking, but it's not always the
   safest option. That said, it's good to be conscious of
   when you're masking, so you can go easy on yourself if
   you're struggling. Tick the examples of masking below
   that apply to you:

   ☐ Suppressing movement and stims.

   ☐ Holding eye contact when it's deeply uncomfortable.

   ☐ Monitoring your body language to make sure it's
   'appropriate'.

   ☐ Hyper-analysing your communication to make sure it
   doesn't come off as 'rude'.

   ☐ Scripting conversations ahead of time.

   ☐ Squashing or minimising your passionate interests.

   ☐ Copying other people's expressions or body language.

Ignoring sensory sensitivities (leading to stress/anger/exhaustion).

Chapter 7: Grief and Burnout

1. Do you have any anger surrounding your neurodivergence? (Honestly, given the way society treats ND people, it'd be almost more surprising if your answer was a straight-up 'no'.) Example: Perhaps you hold some resentment towards your parents/caregivers for not recognising it sooner.

    ....

    ....

    ....

2. If you answered 'yes' to the above, is your anger – or grief – more about the people around you, or wider society and its expectations? Example: Are you feeling frustrated that most workplaces don't accommodate your needs as standard?

    ....

    ....

    ....

3. At times we've felt a lot of sadness – even towards ourselves – usually because we're feeling depleted of energy when it comes to participating in a society that makes it really hard for us. If you have any similar feelings, we think it's healthy to acknowledge them, particularly with a lens that shines a light on how capitalism's expectations are deeply difficult for anyone to attain. This might also be a topic to share with a safe human in your life if you have one (because sometimes you just need to be metaphorically held, right?). Example: Do you wish it was easier for you to hold down a job?

    ....

    ....

    ....

4. Are there any frustrations you need to vent regarding what could've been? Example: Perhaps a relationship ended when you didn't have the understanding you have now. Perhaps you lost a job.

    ....

    ....

    ....

5. If burnout is something you experience, are you aware of the things that can help comfort you? Often we just need to ... PAUSE. But the reality is that this isn't always doable for everyone (horrific, we know). We find ourselves reaching for low sensory environments, extra stimming and food with minimal steps, and putting our egos aside and accepting any help on offer. Example: Maybe stepping away from social media or spending time outside with loved ones (or alone) will help you.

   ....

   ....

   ....

6. Can you think of some minimal, intentional stock phrases that explain your situation, your current energy levels and what you can and can't commit to right now, to help make communication a little easier while you try to recover? Examples: 'Hey, I just wanted to check in and let you know that I'm not intentionally being quiet, I'm just feeling pretty overwhelmed and exhausted and am trying to work through it.'/'Hey, I'm currently feeling pretty burnt out and could really do with any questions or requests being extra specific if that's okay? I'd be super grateful!'/'Hey, just a reminder that I love and appreciate you, even when I'm low on energy and can't show you in the way I'd like to.'

   ....

   ....

   ....

THE PART 2 WORKBOOK 163

7. Are there any signs that tend to arise before you hit the point of complete, unreturnable exhaustion? Are there any responsibilities you can drop if it gets to that point? Are there any standards you can lower so you can be a little gentler with yourself? Example: Perhaps you notice higher levels of anxiety, or struggle to stay in contact with loved ones.

    ....

    ....

    ....

Chapter 8: Dealing with the Fallout

1. Feeling exhausted for an extended period of time after a big realisation is understandable. Have you noticed yourself feeling less able to do things as easily as you could **before** your realisation? Example: Perhaps you are finding your job more difficult post-realisation, or maybe communicating is feeling more taxing.

    ....

    ....

    ....

2. For a lot of late-realised people, something significant happens that makes you realise that something isn't 'right' and prompts the beginning of your journey. This can, quite obviously, be stressful and sometimes force you to re-evaluate circumstances or even relationships around you. Has this impacted any parts of your immediate surroundings, or maybe even changed the way you look at people? Example: Perhaps a relationship came to an end, or you got let go from a job. Or maybe a significant health issue came to light.

    ....

    ....

    ....

3. What does your support network look like? Do you need more support than you're currently getting? Example: Are you able to ask for more help with chores at home? Do you need to ask for deadline extensions, or extra flexibility at work? Do you need to find an online community that makes you feel seen/connects you to people who get it?

    ....

    ....

    ....

4. How has this realisation impacted your mental health?
   Use the scale below to think about how you feel on a
   good day at the moment versus on a bad day:

 1: My absolute lowest, didn't manage to get
out of bed today

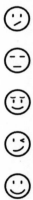 **10:** Felt my best, achieved everything I wanted
to and felt mentally in a good place

5. Since this stuff took a big toll on our mental health, let's touch on coping mechanisms. Write down the ones that work for you, so you can revert back to them if you need to. Example: Finding a community of 'safe people' online (or in person).

....

....

....

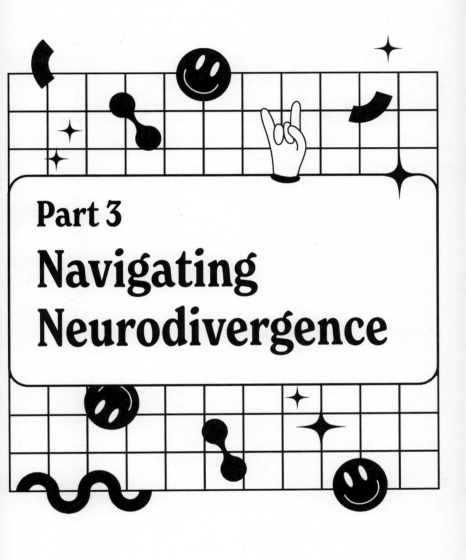

Part 3
Navigating Neurodivergence

Adapt and Adjust

You've gone through a lot of shit, but hope is on the horizon: you've now got the chance to **craft a different life for yourself**. Armed with the knowledge that your brain is maybe a little spicier than others means that you can adapt areas of your life to make them a little easier to deal with.

We hope you know by now that we're not for a second suggesting that it's all on you to push for the changes you need to happily navigate the world with ADHD or autism. Society disables us, and you deserve more than having to spend **all** of your extra energy making up for a lack of help. That's why, throughout this section, we've included how the world should change to accommodate our needs (hey, ya never know who'll pick up this book!).

But it **is** okay to be honest about the things you **do** struggle with. We're not going to lie, friends, this is hard. It can (and probably will) be pretty uncomfortable, but sustainable change doesn't happen overnight. At times it can feel like you've had a total personality and lifestyle overhaul. We've often felt as though, by living in a way that works for us for the first time ever, we're learning to walk all over again.

As you start to make these adjustments and ask for accommo-dations, those around you may also struggle with the 'new' you – but remember, you're not doing it for **them**, you're doing it for **you**. We'll be breaking this section down into all the different areas of your life, so you can skip to the part that you need the most. And please, as you proceed, try to be gentle with yourself. Contrary to what your brain might be telling you, you don't have to change everything all at once.

Are you ready to heal? We've got you.

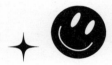

CHAPTER 9

School and University

⚡ **The challenges of education**
⚡ **Asking for adjustments**
⚡ **Our experience of education**

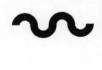

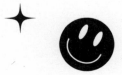

We can't hop in a time machine and go back to school (although that doesn't stop us embracing the joy of glitter gel pens ...), but we can tell you about our experiences of navigating these tricksy places as people with ADHD and autism, and offer you some advice on how to make them work better for **you**.

Why Are Educational Settings So Damn Hard?

When we were at school, ADHD and autism were connected to the stereotype of the disruptive young boy, so our struggles flew under the radar. In fact, young girls were sat next to young boys by teachers to try to get them to cooperate and engage, with no regard for the needs of girls. Because the diagnostic criteria didn't reflect girls' experiences as children (and adults), our needs (and the needs of anyone who sits outside that stereotype) were missed. If we're not getting the help we need now, we definitely weren't getting it then.

School was tough for lots of reasons, many of which you might recognise. The constant skipping between subjects was jarring. As we now know, task switching for autistics and ADHDers is difficult, so our brains don't like being yanked away from one subject and thrown into another. Plus, there were sensory difficulties similar to those we experience in work environments: bright lights, bells ringing, terrible, itchy uniforms – you get the picture.

As we discussed in Chapter 2, sometimes ADHD characteristics are more socially acceptable than those associated with being autistic. A lot of things people categorise as 'weird', such as not making eye contact or repetitive physical behaviours (stimming), are autistic traits, which can mean autistic children are bullied or made to feel like outsiders by their peers.

There's also the non-negotiable fact that neurodivergent brains learn differently to neurotypical brains, and if you haven't got a diagnosis and don't know you have autism or ADHD then you're not going to be learning in a way that's optimal for you.

HOWEVER, compared to the university environments that followed, there was a lot about school that made life easier for our undiagnosed and unrealised neurodivergent brains. At school, our time was largely managed by other people. Our schedules were decided for us, food was provided in the canteen at a certain time, homework had clear deadlines, and pastoral staff were responsible for the wellbeing of the school community. Once we reached university and had to live more independently, all of those safety nets disappeared.

At university, there is a lack of proactive support. It is usually only available if you know about it, and know how to access it, which is great if you're in the situation we are now, but we didn't have the knowledge or self-understanding when we were actually at university to seek out, access and make use of any autism or ADHD support that might have been available. Managing independent life and study was a culture shock. At university, nothing is mandatory and there are fewer immediate consequences if you don't do things. There is so much about university life that seems to work against neurodivergent brains. For example, lectures themselves are delivered in a way that is difficult for monotropic minds to process. Imagine a typical lecture and you'll see that the student is required to do all of these things at the same time:

Listen to the lecture, process the words, view the slides or presentation, write notes (that make sense!) and turn the pages of their own notebook.

This set-up is designed for a polytropic mind, which can look at multiple subjects or tasks at the same time, rather than our minds, which are prone to monotropism and therefore prefer focusing our attention deeply on one thing. This is just one example of the way in which university life doesn't work for brains like ours ...

It's hardly surprising that autistic people are 10 times more likely to drop out of university.[1]

When you think about it, university is **hell** for those of us with neurodiverse brains. (Or at least for some of us, as, hey, we're all different.) You're often thrown into a brand-new situation (tricky) with brand-new people, all with different and sometimes hard-to-understand social cues (trickier), and then, on top of all of that, you're grappling with deadlines and a whole load of information being thrown at you, often in a way that your brain struggles to process. It's total cognitive overload, right?

A 2023 report by student support organisation Unite Students entitled 'An Asset, Not a Problem: Meeting the Needs of Neurodivergent Students'[2] highlighted some of the ways you might struggle in a university environment:

⚡ **Making friends …** You're thrown into this environment and meeting so many different people, some of whom will just not be your sort of people AT ALL (and who, in a halls environment, you're expected to live with!). They may struggle to understand you and that can be tough, particularly for those of us who are carrying trauma or shame from our school days for being different.

⚡ **Sensory overload …** Dim the lights, please! From halls and their noise overload to lecture rooms and their bright lighting, there are a **lot** of sensory issues to navigate, depending on your particular preference and how your brain works.

⚡ **The workload …** A lot of university tasks are built around traditional systems with lots of deadlines and exams, and tutors may struggle to understand that you can do the work, it's just you might need help to deliver it in a different way.

⚡ **A lack of understanding …** We know that we have specific needs that will make our experience so much easier to navigate, such as a quiet room to study in or additional technology to communicate with. But because of the 'hidden' nature of our disability and a total lack of understanding that, yes, it can look this way, it can mean we're labelled as 'difficult' when we simply want to have our needs met.

⚡ **Lack of mental health support …** This is an underfunded area, well, everywhere, but it can also be hard to access it in university, a time when anxiety and depression have been known to rear their mean old heads, particularly in neurodiverse students.

Ugh, there's so much more we could cover here and it's enough to make you think, 'Fuck it, I won't bother.' But the good news is that conversations are opening up around this, research is being done into how to make university environments much more accessible AND it's your legal right to ask for reasonable accommodations at university and at work (more on that later – see Chapter 10), so there are ways to make your experience so much better. We promise.

Mia on ... university

As I mentioned in Chapter 1, university was the beginning of a series of shit life events that I'm still recovering from. Looking back, armed with the knowledge I have about myself now, it's no wonder I struggled.

A big part of my course involved going into the design studio – a place I am now convinced was designed by an evil mastermind to torture autistics. It was so open-plan that you could hear someone eating their lunch from across the room. The lights were bright, overhead and so glaring, and there was nowhere to get any peace. The communal desks were in the middle of the room, so people were constantly walking behind me and if I needed to speak to anyone it would **always** turn into a group conversation. It meant I probably had a grand total of four conversations the entire time I was there! In short, it was a nightmare.

I'd sit in lectures, desperately trying to 'actively listen' and process what was being said. I'd scribble down notes, knowing that if I didn't, I wouldn't remember what was being said, then

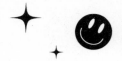

be asked a question. I'd always go blank. It looked like I wasn't listening! But I was. It was just hard for me to compute what was being said. I'd listen to these talks and assume by the end that I'd know what I needed to know. But I'd leave none the wiser, looking around and realising that everyone else got it. At first, I'd ask questions … but after a while I worried that my lecturers would think I was lazy and not listening. So I'd go away and try, pouring hours of work into a project, only to find out later that I had misread the brief and interpreted it wrong.

The mix of not understanding paired with the level of independent study and motivation that was expected hit me **hard**. I was suddenly expected to be able to manage, organise and prioritise without any structure. I could see my peers networking, asking questions and working with the lecturers. But I struggled with this. I was on an isolated island of confusion. Struggling with time management and poor organisation meant I was often late and would walk into a room and sit at the back. I was then way too anxious and embarrassed to speak up and ask questions. It was a vicious cycle.

Some of the most productive and creative sessions I had at university were after 7 p.m. in my tiny halls room with Jess, where we'd turn off the lights, lock the door, light a candle and just sit surrounded by our favourite snacks. Suddenly everything that made focusing difficult disappeared and we could just concentrate on studying in a way that worked for us.

At the end of my second year, I was told that there was no way I was going to pass. I didn't have enough money or energy to repeat the year, so … I dropped out. Perhaps if I'd understood the adjustments I needed in order to work effectively then I would've left university a little less traumatised by the thought of education. Instead, I had a shitload of debt and no self-confidence. The shame attached to failing haunted me for a long time afterwards. I'd always done well at school and I didn't want to drop out; it was just that I had struggled for so long and there wasn't really any way to catch up.

How to Ask for Adjustments at University

We spoke to Tim Dickinson, senior lecturer in education and staff development at Arts University Plymouth (who put support in place for Jess while she was at university), about how best to ask for adjustments to make university life easier for you and your wonderful, spicy brain ...

First of all, remember: it's okay if you're struggling

'A lot of universities and academic institutions are stuck in a traditional idea of how students should deliver their work. There's such a focus on papers being properly referenced, or projects being delivered in front of whole classrooms. These things can be tough for neurodiverse students to do, but in reality there's no need for every student to have to deliver their work in this set, rigid way. I understand that many lecturers are afraid of change and trying new things, in case they go wrong and lose face in front of their class, but there's no shame in a lecturer coming up with a solution that's more adaptable and saying, "Let's give this a go, and if it doesn't work out, we'll still learn from it."'

It's the work you deliver, not how you deliver it, that matters

'The learning outcome can be achieved in different ways. Every student is different. For example, a presentation in front of 250 students might be absolutely breezy for one, but another would be deeply distressed by the idea. If you deliver the presentation, and the ideas within it correctly, it shouldn't matter how that's done. There needs to be more elasticity in how work is both taught and delivered, and it's okay to ask for something that could help you achieve the goal that has been set. **Colleges and universities have a legal requirement to try to remove the barriers you face in education due to a disability. This is known as a "reasonable adjustment".**'

There are lots of ways to adjust

'An example of a reasonable adjustment might be the member of staff sending out the slides used in the lecture ahead of time. This could really help a neurodiverse student feel prepared for what to expect when coming into their lesson. However, many universities struggle to decide what is reasonable and there's no set rules when it comes to this, as it will differ depending on the university and the subject. Your tutor alone shouldn't decide what is and isn't reasonable; that decision should be made collaboratively with the tutor, student and learning support team.'

If they're not listening

'If you have needs that are not being met, first, go to your tutor. The ideal scenario after that is that you, your tutor and the college or university's learning support team (every university should have one) should work together on a reasonable adjustment. But if this isn't happening then, first of all, you could go to your subject leader. If they are the barrier then your student union is the next stop.'

Other Examples of Reasonable Adjustments

⚡ Subtitled video lectures.

⚡ Different formats of lectures or course material.

⚡ Equipment or aids, such as specialist computers.

⚡ One-to-one support.

⚡ Accessible rooms or venues, including quiet spaces.

Jess on ... university

Both Mia and I have always known, due to the way women are socialised, what's expected or needed of us in either work or social situations. This means we could go to parties (but then escape to the smoking area) and we would mask, so we'd be seen to be having a nice time and making friends, when internally we were really struggling. So, as we began to make tiny changes to our lives in university that brought small comforts, people would notice and question (or mock) it. I had nicknames that revolved around me being 'grumpy' and people always said to us, 'You need to get out and make new friends!' But we didn't want to. Find the energy to go out and **talk** to strangers?! I barely had enough energy to keep myself fed and dressed.

It wasn't exactly clear where the lows were coming from, but, given that depression and anxiety seemed to run in my family and the information I had around mental health seemed to put those things down to 'chemical imbalances' and not much else, I didn't dig much deeper. Thankfully, the uni tutors I communicated these struggles to (including Tim) were super-supportive and gave me plenty of extensions to the deadlines, which helped.

In my third year, I didn't have Mia as she'd left by that point. I was lonely and just wanted it to be over. By the time of graduation, I should have wanted to celebrate, but I was too exhausted to enjoy my achievement. There was no euphoric feeling; I felt numb. And because I'd pushed myself so hard, my lupus was exacerbated. All in all, university was an experience of extreme masking for me, and of pushing myself beyond my limits within a neurotypical framework that, so much of the time, was working against me.

Finding the Words

Now, we know all too well that some people insist on just being – um, what's a polite word to use here ...? – ignorant, and no amount of patient explanation will make them a more compassionate person. But if you want the exact language you need to ask for reasonable adjustments, Tim helped us find the words. Try using these if you find yourself in a difficult situation at university:

⚡ 'I find it overwhelming when I arrive to a lecture totally unprepared for what's going to be taught. Would it be possible to send across the slides a day in advance, so I know what to expect when I arrive?'

⚡ 'When you give me feedback it is in big chunks of copy, and I find that too much to process. Would it be possible to receive my feedback in bullet-point form?'

⚡ 'I'm full of dread about doing the presentation in front of all the students, and this is resulting in me avoiding the work. Would it be possible to do the presentation just in front of you and a few others from the class afterwards?'

⚡ 'I can't focus within the studio space – it is too noisy. Would it be possible to work somewhere quieter?'

We know, progress can't come quickly enough, but hopefully the advice in this chapter has given you the tools to advocate for yourself and ask for the accommodations you need – you've got this!

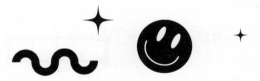

CHAPTER 10

Work

⚡ **Why standard work environments can be difficult for us**

⚡ **How employers can help**

⚡ **Finding your way of working**

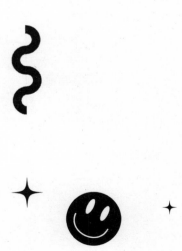

Just as we found university difficult, things only intensified as we moved into the world of work. But a string of subsequent work 'failures' (psst, we didn't fail, we were failed) gave us the tools to see how traditional working environments are set up almost in direct opposition to what neurodivergent brains need, and to forge a different path for ourselves. Let us tell you, besties, this is probably the area of our lives where things have changed the most.

The Problem with Traditional Workplaces

As you're about to find out, we haven't been treated brilliantly when working in corporate environments. It felt, for a long time, that no matter how hard we worked, or how much we justified ourselves, or tried to force ourselves to work like others around us, we wouldn't be seen as good enough in the eyes of our colleagues. And we're not alone – a staggering 30–40 per cent of neurodivergent people in the UK are unemployed;[1] compare that to the national rate, which is currently 4 per cent.[2]

We live in a capitalist society that values our ability to generate profit over who we are as people. When we're at work, we're often in circumstances where decisions are dictated by neuro-typical people with no regard for their neurodivergent employees (and there's usually not a lot of diversity in senior roles, so very little thought is given to the idea that not everyone works in the same way). This means that sometimes we're seen as being not 'productive' enough and therefore valued less in a capitalist system. Ugh.

There are an overwhelming number of factors that make traditional workplaces and expectations hard to manage for neurodivergent brains. Here are just a few (and we **know** you'll have more of your own):

- ⚡ **Sending emails:** When should I reply? How should I introduce it? What tone am I supposed to use? How formal am I supposed to be? Although this is something that people who aren't neurodivergent might consider regularly, too, sending and responding to emails is often a severely anxiety-inducing task for people who struggle with focus and fixate on infinite details.
- ⚡ **Task transitions:** If you're juggling different clients or projects, or have various responsibilities (which, let's face it, most of us do), it can be really difficult to immerse ourselves in one topic and then be expected to switch to something totally different.
- ⚡ **Interacting with colleagues:** It takes energy! Masking is often exhausting, which is why so many of us favour working from home. Pair that with often apologising for things neurotypical society holds against us and we're not even left with that much energy for the job itself!
- ⚡ **Physical environments:** When we're working from home, it allows us to tailor our environment to suit our needs. This might look like dimmed/ambient lighting, a

particular scent and a temperature that works for us, as, while being too hot or too cold isn't particularly nice for anyone, the effect is often reported to be amplified for autistic people.

⚡ **Routine:** While many autistic people do favour routines, it's often not what you think routine is. Managing to get up, get showered, get dressed, feed ourselves and get ready includes many transitions that can be tiring for autistic people. Sure, we might like to do things in a certain way or order, but managing to start a job early in the day and take care of ourselves beforehand is something so many of us feel exhausted by.

⚡ **Sensory experiences:** Given that the majority of workwear doesn't prioritise comfort, sensory issues might also be a struggle for some autistics. Many of us also find that public transport takes a significant amount of energy out of us due to unfamiliar and intense sounds or smells.

Before we started I Am Paying Attention and became self-employed, we worked in a range of corporate environments where we suffered with all of these issues at one point or another. What follows might not make for happy reading, particularly if you recognise your own experience in our stories, but there's light coming at the end of the tunnel, we promise.

Mia on ... work

After leaving university at the end of my second year, I had to find a job – and fast. I was degreeless, penniless and moving back home to face the brutal reality of adult life and I was still unrealised, operating in survival mode. Perfect!

I worked in a bunch of retail jobs to make money while building my design portfolio on the side. I worked my ass off and it was this that got me into the design world. Then, once I was in, I was working 10 times harder than everybody else because I felt inferior. This extreme way of working suited me, as a coping mechanism, for quite a few years until it all completely fell apart. I actively avoided letting anyone know I had failed uni for a long time. It was only when I learnt the stats around just how many autistic students drop out of university education that the shame I carried morphed into frustration at the education system, and sadness for the thousands of students who have been, and continue to be, failed by it.

Even when I was working in corporate design jobs I was still getting to work creatively. That's what I love. The problem was that so many of my jobs were so focused on 'energy'. I need gentle starts, then I can slowly build up to being able to be 'on'. I'd be criticised for not looking totally alert, or for having my video off in calls. For a huge part of the role I felt as if I had to be an actor. I'd have six cups of coffee to be able to look 'alert' and then be impulsive and erratic by lunch.

I kept pushing, though, because for a long time I tied my identity around what I do. I still do that a little; I'm a creative person and that's a big part of who I am. But I'd also tell myself I was 'an ambitious girl' and that's who I was. It led me to overwork, pushing myself to the brink. Even when we launched I Am Paying Attention, I struggled not to work all hours. In those first few weeks I got so much done, but at points I ended up so burnt out I couldn't speak.

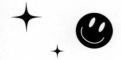

A big wake-up call hit me when my mum fell ill. My mum raised me and my sister as a single mum and she always had a couple of jobs on the go alongside various creative ventures. But that all came to a grinding halt a few years ago when she ended up in hospital. Doctors had very little insight and information initially, and she spent nearly two years fighting for a diagnosis. She now has a functional neurological disorder (FND) diagnosis and struggles with speech on bad days and sometimes relies on mobility devices. Basically, there's a problem with how the brain receives information and sends it to the rest of the body. I know this is an extreme case, but it was a shock for me as I had, up until that point, been living my life very like her. My mum worked as an artist for years. I admired her for how much she was always working, and I replicated it. But I realised that I couldn't just keep going and going and expect my body to be able to cope with it. I knew that if I didn't start saying no, my body would start saying no on my behalf. I'm now searching for balance, as I'm not someone who can relax easily. I'm getting there ... and it helps working with Jess. I've never had a colleague tell me to stop working before! To give you a sense of our career journeys, Jess and I will now share our CVs. Only, unlike in a real CV, they won't gloss over the shitty parts ...

Mia's CV

Duo Boots (as it was called then)

Sales Assistant, 2015. Left because I got let go.

I met some of the kindest, most patient people whilst working in this job, many of whom I still love to this day. But that's the silver lining of an otherwise difficult experience: I wasn't sleeping well so missed shifts, I missed buses, I forgot I'd been assigned shifts so turned up for the wrong ones. Generally, I was pretty unreliable. Nonetheless, I tried desperately to make it work. It took more energy than I had, and the mask was fully on. As soon as it came off at the end of the day, the feeling of mental exhaustion was too much for me to manage. This was definitely a time period where I remember relying a lot on alcohol to unwind, which went about as well as you'd expect. I feel that if I'd known I was autistic and had ADHD at this point, the team really would have been supportive. Unfortunately I didn't, and the burnout and unhealthy coping mechanisms soon caught up with me.

Half Moon Bay

Junior Designer, 2016–2017. Left because I got let go.

This job was probably as far from what I could realistically manage as it possibly could be.

My immediate co-workers were all wonderful (and they probably helped me more than they should have). The pressure started from the moment I began my interview; the bad cop/good cop strategy employed by my interviewers meant that I basically sweated through my entire outfit.

From the sheer sensory overload when I attended trade shows to the anxiety of simply going into the office, I wouldn't be surprised if they considered me one of the worst employees they ever decided to hire. You know what? I thought I was too for WAY too long. But when I look at my current reality and my work environment now, how much I've thrived, and the fact my skills have drastically improved. I'm not so sure that that's true.

We are Jago

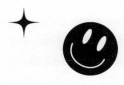

Senior Designer, 2018–2020.
Left because I got let go.

My job at We Are Jago was more complex than other roles I'd had before. I was given more responsibility, more opportunities to build my skills and develop both personally and professionally. I can honestly say that a lot of the skills I've refined while building I Am Paying Attention are ones I picked up from this job.

It was a pretty small team, and to this day I'm still grateful for the opportunity. I was always encouraged and pushed out of my comfort zone, but because I still hadn't had my realisation, the pressure of daily demands started to mount up, and my mental health started taking a hit. My boss would frequently take me to one side and we'd have really constructive talks about how it was going, but it didn't change the fact that I just didn't know how to work with my brain, and trying left me in a state of despair. Eventually, I was let go.

Later, I reached out to my ex-boss I asked him about my time at the company and what made me a bad employee: 'You were never a bad employee, but it was hard to help you properly when we didn't know what you needed ...'

What made me a good employee? 'The excitement of your creativity and your fun, free spirited attitude is what made you special. And the deep conversations that often went off on a tangent.'

Having this conversation gave me some closure and I try not to hold any resentment about my time working for other companies. Because I didn't know about my autism or ADHD, it was hard for me to articulate my needs, which made it hard for my bosses to meet them.

I wanna say it's fucking wild that a) you had to leave university because you couldn't produce work in the way it was being demanded of you, and b) you had to work harder because of that, and c) you had to work even harder because, again, corporate life also fails to accommodate us, and d) you managed to become such an incredible designer despite all of that. You're a design wizard and I'm so proud of you. **- Jess**

Jess on ... work

When I graduated and began to seek out work I didn't know the best ways of working. There was a long period of being hired, then being fired, or leaving jobs as I couldn't 'hack' the pace. Of course, now I realise that, had provisions been put in place for me, things would have looked different. But I will say that all these experiences, however awful, taught me a lot about myself.

Jess's CV

LUSH

Sales Assistant (aka the 'HI, HOW'RE YOU? HOW CAN I HELP YOU TODAY?' girlie), 2015. Left to pursue Salaried Adult Job.

I knew I was good at talking to people; I'd mirror their body language with no problem, and I'd be praised for the 'energy' I was able to bring to the shop floor. I was asked to familiarise myself with the ingredients in the products as 'homework' and I took that literally in a way that I'm **not** entirely sure other people did. That's one thing I've learnt about myself: if someone tells me to do something, I'll take it super-literally. That task in my mind can only be completed if done extremely, extremely thoroughly ... When I'm sure others can skim read and discount the information they won't need, I take it all in, causing total overload.

The Vegan Society

Business Development, 2015–2019. Left as I moved and could no longer hack the two-hour daily commute.

I first started as a volunteer in membership, as I knew I needed a way into a more stable job, and eventually I was hired when a role in business development came up. This was my first job in an office setting, and also the place where I remember the reality hitting that my focus issues were a bit of a problem. I wouldn't ever go so far as to address why I couldn't get work done like everyone else could, but it was obvious enough for me to be constantly stressed and anxious – even outside of work. The feelings of inadequacy were always in the background, and my feelings of self-doubt were regularly confirmed in one-to-one meetings with my managers, as it was said, in one way or another, that I was 'underperforming'.

Thankfully, the role was in the charity sector, and some of the people I met there were an incredible support, reminding me of my strengths and also the reality that I often wasn't receiving enough training. Two of the people in particular who got me through the stresses of that role happen to be incredibly close friends of mine now, and both of them are also late-realised autistics. Surprise, surprise! When I say we're like magnets, I mean it. I'm certain I have some internal radar that seeks out people with brains like mine, because I've accidentally filled my life with people who share plenty of my experiences.

British Pregnancy Advisory Service (BPAS)

Learning and Development Admin Assistant, 2019–2020. Left because I was let go.

It was this role that led me to breaking point. It was my job to coordinate the training for all the nurses and practitioners. Looking back, it's laughable that I thought that role could work for me. There was a lot going on in the company, and while I ended up getting fired from the role, I also helped point out areas where improvements could be made. And while at the time I felt horrendous losing the job, it ultimately did lead to where I am today (but more on that later in the chapter).

I've found confidence in who I am, and accepted that I do have a lot to offer, despite all these difficulties. A big part of reaching this point has meant recognising that working as part of a capitalist system, that values profit above people, is a trap for neurodivergent people. Escaping from it was the best career decision I ever made. If I'd continued to try to adhere to the standards that capitalism demanded of me, I'd have broken down. I am disabled. Capitalism would see me as a write-off, and I know categorically that's not who I am; I have so much to offer regardless of whether I'm able to earn money.

I often can't believe the things you have managed to achieve with ongoing health issues while not getting the support you need. It makes me so happy that we have both been able to create an environment where we are able to properly support each other. I feel so fortunate every day to work alongside someone so thoughtful, creative and empathetic, and it really sucks that so many past jobs weren't able to value this. - **Mia**

Making Work Work for YOU

We became self-employed after founding I Am Paying Attention in 2020. Now, each day we wake up knowing that we can be creative and fun, and we can help people. That we've designed a working life that works for **us** after years of feeling like square pegs in round holes in our old corporate jobs. But going freelance and becoming your own boss isn't possible for (or even wanted by) everyone, so we've also got plenty of tips on navigating traditional jobs.

We know that not everyone is lucky enough to work for themselves **or** able to work with their best friend. But since launching I Am Paying Attention, we've leaned in to a new working style that we think everyone could benefit from. Yes, that includes you, even if you're employed. Hell, it includes those employing you. And even though we don't work this way in order to grind,

grind, grind and be AS PRODUCTIVE AS POSSIBLE, we have found we do get way more done than before, when we were trying to squash ourselves into a corporate way of working.

How we work now

- ⚡ **We're not too hard on ourselves:** Without oversimplifying a very serious problem, at the root of it is that we're now set on being as gentle and kind to ourselves as we possibly can be. At the beginning of every morning, before we do any work at all, we check in with each other, gauge how we're feeling.
- ⚡ **We decide what sort of work we will do that day.** Will we do something light, like make a silly meme? Something that will result in lots of engagement but perhaps isn't too taxing? Or do we feel social, able to send emails and have video calls? Or perhaps we're really wanting to go into deep focus mode and research a topic? There's zero expectation.
- ⚡ **We don't ridicule each other for tripping up.** That happened a lot in our old jobs; we'd get teased if we couldn't do things in a certain way – if we couldn't handle an Excel spreadsheet, for example – when all it would have taken was our bosses giving us 10 minutes to figure out a different way of approaching a task. We found there wasn't much opportunity to reframe in our old jobs; we would be ridiculed for not being able to understand a task in the exact way it was presented to us. Even when writing this book, we struggled with reading these words in one big black-and-white document, so we'd make the text different colours, or make the background pastel. That

way, it'd be far easier to write and digest. We did what we needed to do to make work **work** for us.

⚡ **We swap tasks a lot.** At first, we struggled with this. We were so used to working in environments that were entirely focused on getting things done individually. But now we realise it's okay to rely on each other. It's also okay if there are some things we aren't good at. We don't have to be brilliant at every single little fucking thing.

⚡ **We're each other's biggest cheerleaders.** We'll big each other up constantly – something we both needed when we started, as our confidence levels were truly at rock bottom. We remind each other how brilliantly we're doing. And we make sure to remind each other that we're people before we are workers. If we don't get something done that day, that's okay. Our worth is not defined by our productivity.

What You Can Do ...

We became self-employed to get our needs met at work, but that's just not possible for everyone. If you work for a company and are finding it hard, you're not alone – we've been there. The thing is, being neurodivergent isn't a medical condition that comes with a handy prescription that solves the problem. And because we all exhibit different traits, there's no one-size-fits-all solution and no guarantee that even when you do express your needs, they'll be received well.

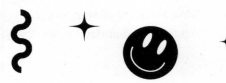

One of the main issues in traditional workplaces is communication. Louise Taylor, a neurodivergent therapist, confirmed that many of her clients have had 'issues' in nine-to-five environments, with colleagues calling them 'odd' or 'rude'. 'My "resting autistic face" is one of confusion, but this can appear to a boss or colleagues as stand-offish or [as if you're] not listening (particularly if you struggle with eye contact),' she says. 'This can lead to being reprimanded for something that you have no control over and is just part of who you are. This can then lead to masking, which we know isn't good for our mental health. Many autistic people can also be quite blunt and the things we say can trigger people, which can lead them to simply attack the trigger (so the person who said it). A large number of working environments are competitive, with a lot of unwritten rules, and often – particularly in my case – I found that I'd either be praised for "saying what everyone else was thinking" or others would be really angry at me for pointing it out.'

We've included our advice for making traditional workplaces work better for you here, but for all the reasons Louise mentions above, take it with a big pinch of 'trust your gut'. If you don't feel safe unmasking in this way, protect yourself first.

⚡ **Find a check-in buddy:** We have each other, and it makes all the difference. If you have a work colleague who you really connect with, each morning grab five minutes with them and chat about how you're feeling. Don't have anyone? Make time to check in with yourself. Sit quietly and ask yourself how you're feeling and what you feel capable of that day.

⚡ **Find your own working style:** Remember, it doesn't have to be how everyone else does it. Some people enjoy setting a timer, removing all distractions and going into hyperfocus. Others, conversely, enjoy switching tasks or sharing problems with a teammate so they're less hyper-independent. Find what works for you.

⚡ **Ask for accommodations:** Remember how we chatted about reasonable adjustments in Chapter 9? They apply in the workplace too, and you have a legal right to ask your employer to help you do your job as well as someone without a disability. If your employer doesn't make these adjustments, this could count as discrimination, and you'd be well within your rights to escalate the complaint. There's lots of useful advice on how to do this on the Citizens Advice website.[3]

When it comes to discussing your need for accommodations and adjustments with colleagues or your boss, it's a lottery as to how you will be received. This is why for a lot of us there's no one-size-fits-all advice. Asking a demanding boss who isn't sympathetic to your particular requirements for accommodations and explaining that you need things done in a different way could lead to those requests being logged and presented to HR as evidence that you're a 'difficult' employee, rather than the boss being identified as someone refusing to put in these accommodations.

There's no 'right' way to do this stuff, but one thing that will make navigating these conversations so much easier is knowing yourself and your communication style, and feeling confident in your abilities. For example, if you begin to recognise that you're often misunderstood by your colleagues or boss, you could preface remarks by saying, 'I don't mean to come across as rude, but this is what I meant.' Showing this kind of self-awareness means you're much more likely to have a productive discussion with mutual understanding.

As tricky as all this can be, we want to be clear, though, that having these conversations can be transformative. As Lia and Sara's stories below show, approaching your manager (and that manager being the good kind) can mean that you're given the accommodations you need to thrive at work.

Lia's Story

Lia, 35, is autistic, and has asked for workplace accommodations that mean she's able to thrive in her job.

I used to be a primary school teacher, and as part of our training we learnt about how autism presents, so that we could identify it in our pupils. There was hardly any material on how it presents in girls, so I set about doing my own research, and began to recognise autistic traits in myself. I used to obsessively collect every single copy of *Vogue* and could recall details from every page; of course, that in itself doesn't mean someone is autistic, but it made me curious.

I went to my GP and she said the things I was experiencing were normal, but I wasn't satisfied. I used my savings to see a private doctor who gave me an autism diagnosis. Being diagnosed helped put some parts of my life into perspective. I was bullied throughout school and considered 'the weird one', and I've also left many jobs. But now I can accept that autism is part of the fabric of who I am and make accommodations for that.

In my old job, working from home wasn't an option, as I had to go to school to teach the kids. I stopped being a primary school teacher, as the environment just wasn't good for me. Of course, the classroom is so busy with different children running around, so sensory issues are really difficult to control.

I retrained as a coder and now work in tech. It suits my brain; I'm obsessed by different languages, and the language of a computer is something entirely new and fascinating to learn. But what has really made the difference is that the company I work for has been willing to meet my accommodations. I disclosed that I was autistic straight away because the HR lead made me feel comfortable. I work the majority of my time from home, unless it's for a social day. My HR lead has done a lot of research into the area, and while my doctor gave me a list of recommended accommodations I could ask for (such as working from home when I need to), nothing is set in stone or rigid. There's a level of understanding and trust there, and as I move and adapt in the job, I can raise things if needed. For example, I recently organised a hackathon for new coders as a way to get more underrepresented people into the business. It was really fun, but my colleagues began to notice me flagging with the social element towards the end. They could see I was becoming drained, so they stepped in and took over the socialising.

I'm not shy talking about my autism and love being able to share with people the things I'm learning. It shows my colleagues there's so many other ways of thinking and being.

Just as Lia did with primary school teaching, Sara has in a role in which she can't work full-time from home. Thankfully, her bosses have been understanding and have made accommodations for her, recognising that getting certain elements of her work done would be easier if they removed distractions from her environment and allowed a work-from-home day when heavy paperwork is needed.

Sara's Story

Sara, 23, works for the NHS on a mental health ward and has found ways to work with her ADHD.

My job involves a lot more than just seeing patients, and it's always been the admin side that I've struggled to keep on top of. I would berate myself for not being able to get my paperwork done in time and would work late into the night trying so hard to get it done and still failing.

Since getting my ADHD diagnosis I've been able to be kinder to myself; if I am not managing to get something done, I tell myself that's okay, go and do another job and revisit it later. My boss has also been incredibly understanding – he's granted me a work-from-home day every fortnight and doesn't pressure me to get my paperwork done before I've had that day. I've also started wearing earplugs during office times when I need to concentrate. I said to my colleagues, 'I can still hear you if you really need me, but they just help me zone out the rest.'

Before my diagnosis, asking for these adjustments would have felt rude, but now I feel like I'm able to work with my ADHD and not against it.

What Employers Should Be Doing to Help Neurodivergent Employees

Most of us have spent YEARS trying to communicate in a way that doesn't work for us, so we think it's about time the rest of society started making some tweaks to their approach, too!

As part of our work running I Am Paying Attention, we deliver workshops to companies and businesses who want to make work easier for their neurodivergent employees, so here are some of the things we tell them (psst, a lot of these things will actually benefit **all** employees):

- ⚡ Respect that we work **differently**, not incorrectly.
- ⚡ Don't leave it to your employee to come to you – be proactive in checking what accommodations your employees need and make sure you're communicating in a style that suits them.

- ⚡ Don't make them feel bad for asking for clarity.
- ⚡ Schedule regular meetings that include more praise than criticism, plus ways to help with obstacles.
- ⚡ Make adjustments to processes (without it being treated like a favour; it's an accommodation, not a fun little treat).
- ⚡ Provide headphones to help us with focus.
- ⚡ Provide accessible software or apps to help with planning. For example, Tiimo is an app that almost gamifies managing tasks in your calendar, which helps to alleviate the anxiety that ND people sometimes have relating to a tight schedule. Notion is a productivity platform that puts everything relating to one project in one place, so we don't have to task-switch so often. Finally, UserWay is a plug-in that we use on our website that makes it accessible by changing the colour and font size for different users.
- ⚡ Praise persistence, not just consistency. We came across an amazing explainer[4] from @adhd_couple that discussed how we, as a society, tend to praise **consistency** – sticking to routines, nailing the exact same 'good' timetable each week (this can apply to all areas of life, including diet and exercise) – but actually **persistence** needs to be praised so much more. Even if your employee doesn't work in a rhythm or stick to something, they're still trying.

REMINDER! ADHD employees can be:

Enthusiastic, hyper-creative, problem solvers, great at adapting, passionate, able to hyperfocus on the things they're excited about, innovative, able to perform under pressure.

REMINDER! Autistic employees can be:

Detail-orientated, driven by efficient ways of working, able to consider problems from many angles, more productive (yes! Research shows autistic employees are up to 140 per cent more productive than their neurotypical colleagues).[5]

Burnout at Work

We talked about how being autistic and ADHD can lead to burnout in Chapter 7, but working in ways that don't serve us can lead to burnout, too. In case you need a refresher, magazine **Psychology Today** reports that autistic burnout is 'a state of physical and mental fatigue, heightened stress, and diminished capacity to manage life skills, sensory input, and/or social interactions, which comes from years of being severely overtaxed by the strain of trying to live up to demands that are out of sync with our needs,'[6] and, of course, a lot of those demands are placed on us in the workplace.

What work-related burnout feels like ...

- Feeding and dressing yourself is even harder than usual.
- Feeling like you have a fraction of the energy you usually do.
- Not even having motivation for the things that interest you.
- Maintaining friendships and relationships outside work is more difficult.

⚡ Making decisions is draining.
⚡ Articulating your thoughts is tiring.
⚡ Extra scattered thoughts.
⚡ Experiencing numbness and dissociation.
⚡ Focusing is harder than usual.
⚡ Getting ready for the day feels unbearable.

There have been very few studies examining autistic burnout in general, never mind in the workplace, but remember Pauline Harley, the wonderful career coach from Parts 1 and 2? A large amount of her work is coaching women through workplace burnout. 'If you've been told all of your life that you're the problem – to the extent that you believe it, too – and you're facing that in work every day and desperately trying to mask your so-called "problems", then it's not surprising this leads to total exhaustion,' she says. This gives us actual chills of recognition. We're expending more energy working in structures and processes that don't work for our brains, which leaves us with an energy deficit. We're always having to work extra hard just to keep our working lives afloat and manage what's expected of us.

'Often, the only way through it is to get out of that toxic environment,' says Pauline. 'We want to encourage autistic people to speak their needs, but that's often not possible when dealing with unresponsive bosses.' Of course, we shouldn't have to quit in order to avoid burnout, but when faced with no other options, it's always better to remove yourself from the situation that's caused you to burn out, with no sign of relief. It's not hard to see why those unemployment stats from page 187 are so high, right?

What You Can Do ...

- ⚡ Embrace the bare minimum and know it's good enough for now.
- ⚡ Wearing pyjamas all day because that's all you can manage? Doesn't make you any less of an adult.
- ⚡ Working from bed rather than your designated working spot? Eating convenience food? It's better than nothing at all!
- ⚡ Explain that you need extra help without feeling bad or apologising. Burnout is hard enough without shaming yourself as well.

Could You Go it Alone?

Abandoning traditional workplace settings is common in our community. A lot of the coaches we spoke to said that their clients often (and sadly not out of choice but because accommodations weren't being met) decided to go their own way and work for themselves. This isn't an option for all professions; there are some jobs (like nursing or teaching, as we heard Lia and Sara talk about on pages 203 and 205) that simply require physically being in a workplace.

But if your career and ambitions do align with being self-employed, we're SO behind you. It will be absolutely no surprise for you to hear that we **love** working for ourselves. That we **love** working together. But it's not all sunshine and rainbows. Here are some of the pros and cons we've encountered along the way:

⚡ **Pro!** It's so much easier to design your working week to suit your needs. You're your own boss and you can be kind to yourself, picking tasks dependent on how you feel that day.

⚡ **Con!** It's really tough to set boundaries for yourself, particularly as, at first, the money worries will be real. We found that we'd set totally unobtainable targets for ourselves and then feel like a total failure if we didn't reach them. Cue overworking in order to feel we'd 'achieved' something. Cue … burnout.

⚡ **Pro!** You decide how jobs get done. Need to work using different colours/apps? In silence or playing loud music? You can make it possible for yourself.

⚡ **Con!** There's a lot of admin involved. Chasing invoices, handling your own finances, etc., and for some of us that can be really tough to manage as our brains simply can't hack the sheer dullness of it all.

⚡ **Pro!** You can fit your schedule around your care needs. If you are someone who needs a lot of sleep, there's no one forcing you to sit at a desk by 9 a.m.

⚡ **Con!** Perhaps it's unfair to call this a con, as really it's just one of life's realities, but you still have to have some structure in place, particularly if others are reliant on you. For example, at the beginning we had to send out a bunch of merch to our customers, but executive dysfunction kicked in and we dawdled on sending those parcels. We felt terrible about that as we knew people had spent their money and wanted their purchases.

⚡ **Pro!** You get to choose who you want to work with and whether they're a good fit for you. When we decide to work with someone, we consider whether we feel like

they'll honour what we need, and respect what we're
good at – and also what we struggle with.

We've said it a thousand times, and we'll say it once more for
those bosses at the back: workplace change can't come soon
enough. Change is hard, we get it. But if you listen and adapt,
everyone will be a lot happier. We're passionate people who
want to pursue careers we love, so when we're forced to behave
in a way that doesn't fit us and operate in offices that weren't
designed for us, and then shamed for not meeting those ideals?
Well, that sucks.

The good news? These conversations are happening. Our
community has shared with us plenty of tales of unaccommo-
dating, stubborn bosses, but they've also told us of bosses and
HR leaders who did listen to them, who recognised that there's
no one-size-fits-all approach to how we neurodiverse individuals work. We see it even with us: what works for Jess won't
necessarily work for Mia. So, when looking into accommodations within the workplace, we're encouraged to see so many
acknowledging that the best thing to do is talk to their ND
employees, listen and make changes based on their feedback.
The more we advocate for our own needs as well as those of
others, the more the message will get through that the people
in charge need to listen.

CHAPTER 11

Family and Friends

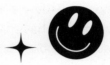

⚡ Navigating family relationships
⚡ Finding friends who understand
⚡ How we socialise now

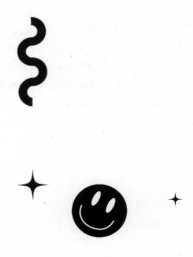

Navigating family relationships and friendship dynamics when you have autism or ADHD or both – whether you're diagnosed or you're still not sure what's going on, and whether those people know what's going on for you or not – is a total headfuck. On the one hand, these are the people who are supposed to love you, who – in theory – know you best. On the other hand, when friends and family deny your experiences because they don't understand them and make some of the stereotypical assumptions we discussed in the earlier chapters, it can be the most painful thing. Ironically, some of the hardest moments you'll experience on your ND journey will be with the people you're closest to.

That said, this journey has seen us discover some new and deeply fulfilling friendships with people who just get it. We have built a support network beyond our friends and families, at the same time as rebuilding fractured relationships within those groups. These relationships have set the bar for the love we deserve. True, wonderful family members and friends can show you how wonderful you are **just** as you are. Along the way, we've learnt a thing or two about how to handle it all, so let's get started …

How to Find Your Way with Family

Obviously, we hope that your family embrace you and your neurodivergence with open arms, but when that doesn't happen, it can be tough. It's possible to evolve beyond friendships that don't work for you, but you can't choose your family, which makes having a family member who doesn't support what you're going through extra-difficult.

In Chapter 10, we met neurodivergent therapist Louise Taylor. She says that when a late diagnosis or realisation comes, we start viewing ourselves and our histories through a new lens. 'You start seeing how much crap you've received from the people you love, what you normalised and what's no longer tolerable, and, in some cases, the ways you were abused for being neurodivergent.' It can be empowering to get to know yourself better, but that can also come with grief. 'You may have to let go of the relationships that no longer serve you, and that does include your family,' she adds.

'I support a lot of people who are deeply traumatised by family systems or family members, those who have reached the point where they cannot be around them, or their family have estranged themselves from them, as they find they cannot accept their child for who they are.'

Louise advises asking yourself these questions:

- ⚡ What is love to you?
- ⚡ Who is cheering for you?
- ⚡ Who makes you feel safe?

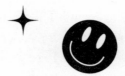

A lot of autistic people are very loyal and will see the good in people, particularly their family. We've both had a lot of experience with this. But, Louise says, you need to allow yourself the space to dig into how they make you feel, because you want to ensure that the majority of your time is spent in healthy, kind and compassionate relationships – and, sometimes, that may not be your family. Ask yourself:

- ⚡ How do you feel in their company?
- ⚡ How do they make you feel? Is it easy? Or draining?

Trust your instinctive answers to these questions. You can acknowledge that you love them and want to spend time with them, but that time might look different to normal; it might involve avoiding certain triggers or limiting how long you spend with them.

But – a caveat: 'I often see that once someone gets a diagnosis, they can then want every wish and accommodation to be met. That's not realistic,' says Louise. Boundaries have to be about keeping **everyone** safe, not just the person who is setting them. And to be able to know your boundaries you really need to know yourself, so you can then go to a family member and say, 'I'm not saying that it's your intention, but it does upset me, and we need to work around this as it's for my health.'

'Try to examine how they could be feeling and whether what you're asking for is achievable,' says Louise. 'The more you're aware of how you come across, the more you can find a balance that suits everyone.'

Jess on ... parents

When I was younger, my mum always said things like, 'I think you might be on the spectrum,' but she didn't go further than that. I suppose what was considered a cause for medical intervention has shifted slightly in recent years.

Now, she feels she let me down by not taking my suspected autism and ADHD more seriously back then, but I think she was going above and beyond to support my needs. She couldn't do enough for me, always validating my emotions and never making me feel as if she didn't accept me, but because she didn't pursue her instincts, I didn't get any support for my neurodivergence at school, for example.

For a while, both Mia and I put early diagnosis on a bit of a pedestal. Sure, there are things that make life easier if you know how you work, but I'm now a lot more comfortable with the idea that there would've been challenges whichever route we took. Ultimately the way society views neurodivergent people is the problem – and those who have a medical diagnosis earlier don't get to escape that by any means. I tell my mum this in the hope that she'll feel less guilty.

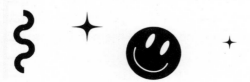

Parental Acceptance

What Jess's story makes clear is that even when family relationships are healthy, a neurodivergence diagnosis or realisation can still be fraught with difficult feelings. Heather Parks, a neurodiverse family coach, agrees that parents can feel a lot of guilt and shame that they haven't recognised neurodivergence in their children (at whatever age). Unlike in Jess's situation, that can sometimes lead to parents resisting acceptance. 'Parents can struggle to understand and separate what is neurodivergence and what are mental, physical, social, emotional and identity issues which may have emerged as a result of their neurodivergence being unknown – or known, but not fully accepted or validated. Growing up without a sense of identity and belonging, where expectations regularly exceed capacity, and where social, sensory and educational environments have not met needs creates chronic stress. And this long-term stress is a huge factor in the neurodivergent person's wellbeing. Parents may have been given different explanations by professionals for why their child was struggling or made their own conclusions. Accepting a new explanation can be hard. Owning that their parenting and their own beliefs and expectations may have contributed to their child's challenges is even harder. Some parents will embrace the new information. Some may experience denial.'

If your parent (or another family member) seems hostile, the next step is – yep, you guessed it – to create boundaries. These can be emotional or time-based. 'It might be deciding to only spend one Sunday afternoon a month with them, for example,' says Heather. 'It's about honouring your own needs without necessarily having to go into that blame, judgement and shaming of other people, because that doesn't actually feel good, either. You could say something along the lines of: "I've noticed that I'm getting very tired recently. I have only a limited social capacity, so for a while I need to just step back."'

The other person might not like it, but it's important to learn to be okay with other people not being okay. 'This is tough, as we may not be used to putting our own needs first and we fear taking any action which may result in any further loss of connection,' says Heather. 'Learning to create boundaries which protect our wellbeing and put our own needs first can feel a little uncomfortable and many need support when they first start to figure out a new dynamic with friends and family.'

Talking to family about autism and ADHD is hard enough, but for some of us there are additional difficulties. Many of you will have to deal with cultural expectations or – as Asia discusses below – will have grown up in fraught or unsafe environments that make it **really** hard to unmask and just be yourself.

Asia's Story

Asia, 22, was diagnosed with ADHD last year after pushing for a diagnosis since she was 17. At first, her mum struggled to accept her diagnosis.

When I was a teenager, my mum suggested I could have ADHD, but back then we weren't getting on. She has bipolar and I thought she was saying it to be cruel to me, to make an excuse for the way she was treating me at the time. We were clashing non-stop. I'd have these outbursts that I couldn't control. I'd yell things that I hadn't even thought about but felt strongly in that moment, saying I hated her. I just couldn't calm myself down and then I'd feel intensely guilty afterwards. With my mum's bipolar and my undiagnosed ADHD there was a lot we were contending with, and we'd spend weeks at loggerheads.

I was also bullied at school and felt like I didn't fit in. I have difficulty with vocal regulation, and I have depression and anxiety, which is really common in people who are undiagnosed; this made it difficult for me to make friends. There were lots of things I'd beat myself up about that I now realise is my ADHD. I'm sad that I didn't get that support I needed when I was younger, but I was eventually diagnosed with ADHD when I was 21. Now, I'm able to recognise some things that I do that aren't neurotypical. The way I see it, my brain is just a bit funky! But the biggest change has been in my relationship with my mum.

She was happy for me when I was finally diagnosed with ADHD. It had taken a long time to get the diagnosis, and she knew how tired I was of not knowing for sure, so having it confirmed both lifted a weight off my shoulders, but also made me really sad that I had suffered for so long without the support I needed. She was frustrated that there wasn't as much information when I was younger that could have shown us how ADHD can present in females; otherwise we might have known sooner.

Now, my mum does so much research that she knows things about my ADHD before I do! We're both better able to understand each other and our needs. But we've had to have a lot of difficult conversations, one of which was about how badly we clashed when I was younger. After the diagnosis, I was able to look back and contemplate how ADHD had affected me and my relationships growing up. Having ADHD explained so many of my difficulties and why my needs and reactions to things were different than expected for someone my age. It was difficult for us to look at it objectively, but finally being able to have an answer as to why I had so many issues growing up left us feeling like we could finally move on.

A lot of my frustrations in my relationship with my mum stemmed from miscommunication, due to both our different perspectives (her black-and-white thinking, and my overanalysing and sensitivities) and our needs being different. But it came from the same place: wanting to understand each other and feel the support we needed from the other person. Now that it is clearer what my needs are and how things can affect me differently – such as environmental stimuli, body language, tone of voice – our relationship in general feels a lot more manageable, especially how I communicate my needs.

For example, earlier today we had the fan on and the TV on, and my mum was chatting at me excitedly, but I was having difficulty managing everything. I felt far too overwhelmed by it all and knew I was close to having a meltdown. Because I was able to identify why I was feeling this way rather quickly, I was able to communicate this and resolve it by asking to turn off the fan. Removing this one environmental stimulus made everything else more manageable.

If anyone was struggling to get a family member to listen to them, I'd advise them to take time to consider their own feelings, and make sure they have time to themselves where they can consider their own needs. Having clarity on that will make communicating with your parents so much easier.

More Questions Than Answers

We don't know exactly what causes autism and ADHD, but both can be genetic. At the moment, many young adults are being diagnosed with both conditions, and those diagnoses (or realisations) are prompting their parents to explore their own possible neurodivergence. This can all make telling your parents about your suspected or confirmed autism or ADHD hella confusing – for you and for them. Hey, it's yet another layer of nuance you may be faced with on this journey.

Are You Masking Without Realising?

As we try to unpick our relationships with friends and family, it can be hard for us to recognise what is masking and what's just us, because so often we've been masking but we didn't know it. Signs that you're doing that include:

⚡ Not processing emotions.
⚡ Forcing eye contact or looking between the eyes.
⚡ Hiding or minimising personal interests.
⚡ Scripting conversations ahead of time.
⚡ Copying expressions or gestures.
⚡ Always thinking of the impression you leave on people.
⚡ Overthinking how to stand or act.
⚡ Monitoring your body language to appear relaxed.
⚡ Suppressing movement and stims.
⚡ Bottling things up to avoid appearing 'too sensitive'.
⚡ Ignoring sensory sensitivities and feeling stressed.

Jess on ... her mum

I mentioned earlier in the chapter that my mum saw not recognising my autism and ADHD as a personal failing. I gave her reassurance that she did what she could with what she had, and I can now see that part of this lack of recognition might have been down to the fact that she's autistic, too. We've always joked that I'm a 'copy and paste' of my mum, and she and I now agree that a lot of my struggles going unnoticed were likely down to

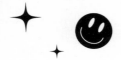

the fact that she could often relate to me deeply, maybe a little more intuitively solving some of my problems for me without realising that they aren't things everyone struggles with – and that might be because she's autistic herself.

Finding Friends Who Understand You

It can feel like there are a lot of unspoken **expectations** when it comes to friendships. You know the ones: you **must** agree to attend the brunch every weekend; you **have** to reply to messages right away; even, you've **gotta** go to a friend's birthday, which, by the way, is gonna be held in a super-crowded, loud bar. There's so much about friendships that can be difficult for autistics and ADHDers, like becoming anxious in social situations, struggling to interpret body language and, yes, meeting friends' (sometimes endless) expectations.

Of course, there's no reason why neurodivergent and neurotypical people can't be friends – in fact, many of our friends are neurotypical. With some, we've been super-lucky and they've just got us straight away. They've recognised what we need. But others, particularly old friends or family, can struggle with the idea that something we were totally **fine** with before (except we weren't fine, we were masking) is not fine anymore. Hello!? Isn't everyone allowed to grow and change?!

True friendships should be about adapting to each other's needs so that you shouldn't have to mask. But to get there you might need to have a few tough conversations with the people you have grown up around. Then, it's about recognising if they're willing to grow and change with you or if they're going to grow away from you.

Mia on ... friendships

When I first arrived in Brighton, I felt like I needed to make friends and got in with a group of girls. I moulded myself into the group, masking constantly, and managed to fit in for a while. But then their expectations started kicking in: I had to be constantly active in our group WhatsApp, bitch about other girls in the circle if they cancelled plans, and always attend brunch dates in our large group, somewhere noisy and bright, making small talk for two or three hours. I felt trapped.

It must have been obvious, because they told me I didn't need to feel anxious about them, but the very idea of being in such a large group setting made me feel so uncomfortable. On one occasion, I was supposed to meet them for lunch and my legs were trembling as I stood at the bus stop because I knew I'd have to snap into a character – that's how much I feared it, hated it. This was pre-realisation, so I didn't have the language to communicate how I was feeling to them or myself. Now I know that I was struggling for a reason.

Some things I find difficult in friendships: I can't deal with goal-posts changing. For example, if I'm invited to go somewhere and I think it's going to be one-on-one and then I arrive and it turns out it's a group hang. Pre-realisation, I used to try to just force myself into these big, buzzy friendship groups. I was so confused as I liked these people; I just got so anxious and stressed being with them. It wasn't them; it was the situations I was putting myself in to please them. I also found replying to messages all the time difficult. It felt like I was good at making friends but struggled to maintain them.

Over the past few years, though, I've got a lot better at recognising my boundaries and communicating them. It's not been easy and, I can't lie, there's been times when I've handled those conversations badly. But I'm not going to beat myself up about that – mistakes are all part of the journey. I've looked back and thought, 'Yes, I could have responded better, but I'm also human.'

I know that not everyone I meet is going to have a brain that works like mine. So, sometimes I will have to educate someone on what works for me. That's become so much easier since getting to know myself better.

Now, I've got some core friends who I only see once or twice a year. Or friends who I can message and say, 'I absolutely love you' and then we'll not speak for a few months. There's no expectation with them, whereas I've had fallouts in the past when people have viewed my behaviours (such as retreating to my phone when I feel overwhelmed) as rude and called me out on that.

For years, masking made me so exhausted and unhappy, and when I had my realisation and began unmasking, some friends found it hard to understand. For them, it was like my entire personality was changing. Some are accepting of that, and some aren't. I understand why it can be hard for people to see someone they love suddenly change their behaviour or the way they navigate relationships. It can be a shock, but it is possible to have these conversations in a sensitive way, so that you prioritise yourself and don't apologise, but you also have compassion for the other person and how they might be feeling.

Jess on ... friendships

I've spent a lot of time figuring out who I should give my energy to, and who I shouldn't. I've realised several times that I was essentially being an unpaid therapist for friends – and that, given that I was getting less energy back in return, it didn't feel mutually beneficial. Don't get me wrong, it's important that I'm there for my friends, but if you, like me, find yourself setting boundaries that are repeatedly being ignored, or someone seems to only want to spend time in your company if it's to talk about **them**, that's probably not a sign of a good friend or someone who deserves access to you all of the time.

Truthfully, I've learnt this the hard way. I need to be surrounded by people who are self-aware enough to recognise when they're asking too much of me. If I need to explain myself over and over and they're not getting it, I'm going to have to call it quits. Unfortunately, being disabled means I have less energy, and I don't want to expend it in the wrong places. I love HARD, but if I do have excess energy, I want to invest it in myself and making my life more comfortable. I have plenty of friendships that serve as reminders that I shouldn't come away from them feeling mentally exhausted, but rather revived. I can't settle for friendships that leave me full of anxiety or stress any more. Let's be real here, sometimes you just have to have a brutally honest conversation with yourself and analyse what's more important:

this person's needs or the fact that you're burning out by continually putting their needs first?

Hey, you! You're an amazing friend!

There are so many things that make neurodivergent people utterly wonderful friends. We can be very passionate and excited about things, and when that's directed at a friend's achievement, that feels **really** special. The same goes for our keenness to understand things from many angles (this is why we'll ask you plenty of **genuine** questions when you're talking). We're super-passionate people and, contrary to the stereotype, we can be hyper-aware of how others are feeling.

The research isn't yet clear on whether these traits are derived from ADHD, autism or both, but the point is that we feel it's unfair if someone accepts all the great parts of being your friend, while holding other elements of your neurodivergence against you.

Let us remind you right now, in friendships:

- ⚡ You shouldn't have to bend yourself into something you're not.
- ⚡ You shouldn't have to exhaust yourself for any relationship.
- ⚡ You are perfect as you are.
- ⚡ Not having the energy to communicate is not something you should feel guilty about.
- ⚡ You should feel comfortable being your authentic self.

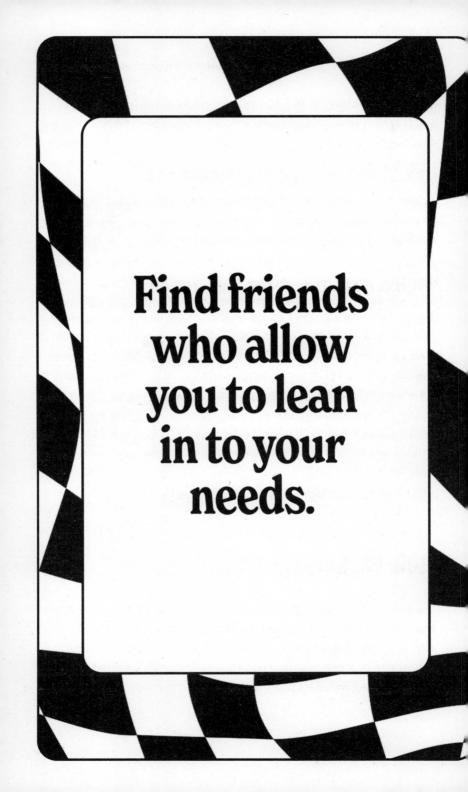

Find friends who allow you to lean in to your needs.

Being able to have those shared experiences and be open with each other, while also listening to their perspective on things, has been life-changing and lifesaving for us. So, we hear you ask, how did you find them? Online! Don't be ashamed to seek out friendships from ADHD and autistic communities online. Some of our very best friends we've never even met in real life! We've listed our favourite online ND besties in the Resources section at the back of the book (see page 339).

Welcome to the sorry-free zone!

By recognising what we can offer as friends and being true to our authentic, unmasked selves, we've managed to build an awesome group of friends, many of whom are autistic or have ADHD. Let us tell you, finding a community of people who innately understand you and your needs is fucking wonderful.

Among us, we call it: THE SORRY-FREE ZONE. Don't want to hang out tonight as you're knackered and had way too much stimulation for the day? Don't say sorry! That's ace. Look after yourself. Prioritise your energy and don't force yourself into a conversation with us.

How We Socialise Now

When we were masking, we'd sometimes try to hide our excited reactions for fear of coming across as immature or 'childlike'. Expressions of genuine thrill aren't always accepted in adults, but in the process of unmasking we've allowed ourselves to let that show. As we've let our masks drop, rediscovering the joy in things that we love but have pretended we don't to avoid seeming immature – such as videogames, going to theme parks or colouring in – has been so healing and has enabled us to be more authentic, better friends.

The same goes for accepting that, as people with autism or ADHD, we need time alone to decompress from social interactions. We live apart but chat and message every day. When we visit each other or travel together, we build in time to ourselves. If we're away, Mia will always go and check out if there's anywhere to swim, while Jess wants to spend time doing her skincare. We allow each other to decompress. We don't see needing to spend time apart as an insult. Everyone has their own needs and we lean into that.

Jess's dream hang

I love being at home with a friend, or maybe two, with fairy lights or mood lighting (not in **that** way, all right?), and just relaxed in each other's company. Also, I like a plan that doesn't involve getting up and going to multiple different places. When I'm having to navigate streets, I'm trying to think where I'm going, not bump into people, tune out loud noises, maybe try to ignore the fact that I'm too cold or hot or struggling with brightness. Sensory overload central. Basically … give me minimal stress. Oh, and somewhere with good snacks. Snacks are necessary.

Mia's dream hang

For Jess, it's all about the sensory stuff. For me, it's about being with the right people. I don't mind bowling or being in busy places as long as I know that the people I'm with are safe people who, if I turned round and said, 'Can we get out of here?' would totally understand and be like, 'Yep, let's go.' I think that's why I find group settings stressful, as there's less flexibility to do that. When I go places with my partner we go at our own pace, in our own little bubble, and make little stops wherever we go. If I go shopping I take it slowly, not going into every shop, and making sure we have plenty of coffee stops.

Thank-you Notes for Those People Who Really Get It

We'd like to say thank you to the people in our lives who let us be us, in all our ND glory:

- ⚡ Thank you for understanding that communication isn't always easy for me when I go quiet.
- ⚡ Thank you for helping me with obstacles.
- ⚡ Thank you for implementing my accommodations and adjustments with kindness and respect.
- ⚡ Thank you for taking time to learn what support looks like for me.
- ⚡ Thank you for advocating for me.
- ⚡ Thank you for being an active part of my healing.

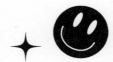

CHAPTER 12

Relationships and Sex

⚡ **How we experience sex**
⚡ **Seeking stimulation**
⚡ **Sexual and gender identity**
⚡ **Navigating relationships**

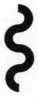

When we first started I Am Paying Attention, we wanted to talk about all of the things that weren't being talked about when it came to ADHD and autism. Sex and relationships were BIG ONES. A lot of neurodivergent people can be infantilised by others, but we're not children; we're fully grown adults. And part of being an adult is entering into relationships with people, having sex and discovering what you like – and don't like. That can be messy, for everyone. Because, let's be honest, these things are hard to unravel whether you're ND or not … Everyone has different love languages, past traumas and experiences of ex partners, and women and LGBTQ+ people also have to decode what shame has been placed on them by our patriarchal culture.

There are so many tricky questions to answer, and it will take some time to work through them all, but the running theme throughout this whole book (and, let's face it, our entire lives) is that getting to know yourself and not feeling like you need to fit in is a brilliant thing. The better we understand ourselves, the easier it is to navigate the tricky shit. Learning about ADHD and autism has really changed our relationships and our sex lives. We are both currently in happy, fulfilling relationships, but that doesn't mean that we think long-term relationships are what **everyone** should be aiming for. We just want you to be able to figure out what happy and content looks like for **you**.

Let's Talk About Sex

First of all, we just want to caveat all this by saying that this is all super-personal. One chapter, and our experiences, cannot cover everything you feel, or what's going on in your mind and body. For one thing, the conversations are always changing. New sexualities and ways to identify are emerging all the time. You also don't have to decide just yet or remain in one 'box' forever. You can sleep with who you want to sleep with, or you can sleep with no one at all. You get to make the rules. 'Sexuality is a personal journey that you should take some time to examine on your own terms,' explains Louise Taylor, the neurodivergent therapist we met earlier. 'What does pleasure mean to you?' She also advises examining what thoughts to do with shame and sexuality might have been instilled in you by other people. 'I grew up in Northern Ireland so can see how much religious indoctrination impacts these things. I was terrified of sex and that's taken years and years of work [to undo].'

There's so much shame to grapple with, not just from religion, but also wound up around how a 'good' or 'bad' woman should behave. We will have internalised that shame and tied it tightly to our own experiences of being neurodivergent. For example, **sensory issues could play a part in whether or not you enjoy sex**. You might only enjoy sex on a certain type of bedding, or sensory stimulation could greatly enhance the experience for you, and you may feel super turned on by someone breathing on you. That's why, at the heart of it all, it's vital to explore your-self and have open and honest conversations with partners about what you like and don't like.

There's also very little discussion or research on this topic, particularly when it comes to women. Even those within our community could be misguided. 'We don't really have an image of female autistic sexuality, as so many of the narratives out there have been written by men,' explains Amy Gravino, a relationship coach and sexuality advocate for the autistic community. 'I've been to so many support groups where I'm the only woman in a room of men. There are also, in general, a lot of myths and misconceptions when it comes to autistic people and sex. One of the main ones I talk about is that autistic people are asexual. There certainly are people in our community who identify as asexual, but it's become the stereotype of our whole community, which isn't correct. Autistic people, like everyone, have and enjoy sex.'

When it comes to dating and trust, however, there's also a risk of learning from the wrong people and being taken advantage of. 'Autistic people are often infantilised. We're told we shouldn't trust our instincts, and this can be taken advantage of,' explains Amy. 'Bullying and feeling ostracised by our peers can also play its part. I was bullied throughout my teen years, so when I reached college I was so broken. It led me to want to trust, and do anything, for people who were nice to me. Many autistic women are not taught what abuse looks like, that it can come in different manifestations, so I come across a lot of women who don't even know that they are being abused. We just normalise it as that's all we know.'

The good news is that the work you do examining your own self, your pleasures and needs, can also be really powerful when it comes to seeking out the good people in your life. 'Being totally authentic and upfront in the dating world about what you want and don't want serves as a really good arsehole filter!' explains Louise Taylor. 'If you ask for what you want and are ghosted, that means they weren't the right person for you.' Finding someone who you can have open and honest communication with around sex is important, as is self-examination (something autistic people are very good at!), to figure out what you like and don't like.

'For me, I also worked on myself from the ground up. The validation I had so desperately craved I managed to find in myself,' says Amy. As with all conversations we've had in this book, looking inwards first puts you in a really strong place to navigate all the complications that come with modern-day dating.

Seeking stimulation

There are a huge number of reasons why a neurodivergent person might find it hard to relax enough to enjoy sex, including:

- ⚡ Sensory overload from the lighting, the bedding or the feeling of someone else's skin.
- ⚡ Struggling with temperature regulation.
- ⚡ If you've masked for a long time, you might not know what your own needs or desires are and therefore find it difficult to communicate these to your sexual partner.
- ⚡ Because many of us don't identify as straight (more on this shortly) but perhaps don't feel entirely clear on our sexuality, we might not be having the sex we want with the person we want. Understanding and articulating that is **hard**.

However, sometimes the opposite is true, and we see sex as a solution for problems that are actually connected to our neuro-divergence. A lot of people in our community look to sex to fulfil a compulsive desire for stimulation, or as a quick-fix, thrill-seeking behaviour. If you recognise yourself in this discussion, you might see yourself in Mia's experience.

Mia on ... sex

If you are related to me in any way then it is illegal to read this! My late teens and early twenties were ... explosive, to say the least. I hadn't had my ADHD and autism realisation yet, and I was in an environment that was loud, noisy and full of people drinking too much, taking drugs and having a lot of sex. When I look back at my memories of that time, they're not fond ones. They make me feel anxious, and for a long time I felt ashamed of myself.

From a very young age I'd get into relationships and then learn that, behind my back, other people were warning the guy I was with about me. Unfortunately, that's not uncommon for any woman who chooses to have multiple partners and explore her sexuality in that way. That shaped an early attachment to shame that only carried on once I got to university. I was using casual sex as a form of stimulation, even above and beyond enjoyment. I became a little bit addicted to how it made me feel, the rush that came with having sex with lots of new people. It would be different if I was having casual sex like that now, but as I was just maturing, I was still trying to get to know myself and what I liked. I still hadn't figured out what was okay and what wasn't.

I've always been so close to Jess, but there were even things that, back then, I wouldn't speak to her about, as the decisions I was making didn't feel aligned with who I was. There was the person I thought I was, and then there was this other version of me who drank a lot and got into situations with people that would stain how I felt about myself for weeks.

Is It Chemical?

Some studies suggest that ADHD could be linked to low levels of a neurotransmitter called dopamine, but we don't yet know enough about how low dopamine actually affects individuals with ADHD. There's no proof that our thrill-seeking behaviours can be directly attributed to a 'lack' of dopamine, and suggesting they are would be simplistic. As Dr Devon Price writes for online platform **Medium**, 'As objective and scientific as neurotransmitter activity **sounds**, we don't currently have a way to actually measure it in patients' brains. If someone exhibits common ADHD traits (trouble keeping track of time, or a cluttered house), there is no biological way to validate the diagnosis by checking their dopamine levels. We aren't even sure if ADHD actually is caused or instantiated by differences in dopamine levels.'[1] What we do know is that when we orgasm, our brains release chemicals including dopamine and oxytocin, and given that ADHD brains are interest-driven and often searching for stimuli to focus on – whether it's healthy or not – it's easy to see how sex might become something that people with ADHD chase. If you have ADHD, feeling under stimulated might feel incredibly unenjoyable. Other ways under-stimulation can show up include:

Irritability, not feeling content, struggling to relax, craving substances, clouded thoughts, difficulty communicating, need to be productive, hyperenergetic movement, anger/frustration, distracted, racing thoughts, feeling anxious, picking/biting, impulsivity

Since we began to recognise that our drinking, picking arguments and having short sexual encounters might be us seeking stimulation, we've noticed that we do these things so much less. We'd love to tell you exactly how to do this and give you the solution, but really it all reverts back to knowing your brain better and understanding that your ADHD or autism means you're wired this way. What we're saying is, none of this is your fault, but by leaning in to what feels comforting and giving yourself a bit of a break when you are struggling, you'll feel better. We asked our community what they did during a bout of feeling under-stimulated, and they said:

- ⚡ Put on a song you love and move your body to it.
- ⚡ Make notes of the things you want to impulse-buy (rather than actually buying them).
- ⚡ Go for walks.
- ⚡ Voice-note friends.
- ⚡ Pick up a book.
- ⚡ Go for a swim.
- ⚡ Sing a song really loudly.
- ⚡ Play a game, or get a fidget toy.

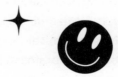

Neurodivergence and Sexual and Gender Identity

We know that, like many other neurodivergent people, we think deeply. If there's an ounce of doubt or an unanswered question, we will go into that from all angles. We do have to remind ourselves that we don't always need defined answers. But, at the same time, we're learning about our brains from scratch and asking ourselves questions that examine what we've been taught since childhood and ripping up the expectations placed on us, so it's understandable that we want them.

Many neurodiverse people also go on a journey of self-discovery when it comes to their gender and sexuality. There's a lot of evidence to show that neurodivergent individuals are significantly more likely to identify as LGBTQIA+ than those who are neurotypical.[2] Take the recent Cambridge study which found that autistic people might be three times as likely to identify as trans, while another study found that neurodivergent individuals were eight times as likely to be asexual.[3] The studies haven't dug into why this could be (something that would be quite impossible to conclude considering how complex and individual gender and sexuality identities are for us all), but the predominate theory is that neurodivergent people have a lesser tendency to follow societal norms. As we said, we are **all** about burning that rule book, which tells us who, and what, we should be.

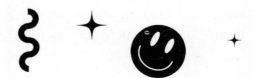

This is where the term 'neuroqueer' comes in, coined by Dr Nick Walker in 2008, who then played with the idea for a few more years before – alongside friends and colleagues Athena Lynn Michaels-Dillon and Remi Yergeau – introducing it into their communities and broader culture in 2014. There are many ways to use the term 'neuroqueer' – as both a verb, an adjective and a label of social identity – and we'd thoroughly recommend you read Dr Nick Walker's book **Neuroqueer Heresies: Notes on the Neurodiversity Paradigm, Autistic Empowerment, and Postnormal Possibilities** to learn about them all. They include being both neurodivergent and queer, with some degree of 'active exploration around how these two aspects of one's being entwine and interact', as well as trying to undo our cultural conditioning and ingrained habits of heteronormativity. 'A neuroqueer individual is any individual whose identity, selfhood, gender performance, and/or neurocognitive style have in some way been shaped by their engagement in practices of neuro-queering, **regardless of what gender, sexual orientation, or style of neurocognitive functioning they may have been born with**,' Walker writes. In fact, to even define the term in an authoritative way kind of defeats the purpose of it, as Walker says: 'The sort of people who identify as neuroqueer and engage in neuroqueering tend to be the sort of people who delight in subverting definitions, concepts, and authority.'[4]

As part of this journey of self-discovery, 'You're calling into question all of these different labels, and whether or how they're right for you,' explains Natalie Roberts, a relationship coach who now identifies as neuroqueer. 'This journey of identity is one we naturally embark on when we discover neurodiversity – in relation to ourselves, our relationship and/or our family. Depending on the support you have around you, it can become an identity revelation and breakthrough or an identity crisis. When my husband found out he is autistic, I read loads about autism and decided I was neurotypical. ADHD wasn't on our radar yet and neurodivergent women wasn't really a thing at all 10 years ago! In my business, coaching individuals and couples in neurodiverse relationships, a huge part of what I support ALL clients to do is reconnect with themselves. Who are they? Who have they been trying to be? What stories have they been told about who they are or should be and what a happy and successful relationship looks like?' More recently, when Natalie's teenage son came out as trans, they began to have open conversations about gender and sexuality, and the result was transformative. 'As I listened to how my son had been experiencing and exploring his identity, I began to wonder again about the "labels" of my own identity and the influence they have on me being me? I've experienced my life as "woma"', as a teen I assumed I'm straight, and with the awareness of neurodiversity in my relationship, I'd decided I'm neurotypical. As I was walking and wondering about all this one day, I had an idea that felt bonkers and liberating at the same time! I decided to ditch those labels for a while and see what happens – no one else knew, only me! I'd done this already with other aspects of me but these had previously felt very fixed to me. It's all an invitation to become aware of the 'maps' of our identity and to evaluate and maybe ditch some or all of those societal norms and rules so that we can find new ones and be true to ourselves ... Identity (including our neuro-identity) belongs to us and it isn't fixed in the way it's presented to us; it becomes labelled and fixed because of the society and culture we live in. Labels may get us somewhere but not everywhere, and maybe not forever. Our identity has often

adapted and squeezed itself into boxes and is actually desperate to be explored inside and then lived out, and also to keep
evolving as we experience more of life and connect with others.
It's liberating to begin this inner work and become more and
more of you! A huge part of my job is engaging with people who
have come through the doorway of neurodiversity and want
support to discover 'Who am I and how do I be me?' As Natalie
explains, and as we've discovered, so much of this stuff is inter-
twined and, at the heart of it, it's good for us all to examine who
we are and why we behave in certain ways. 'There's so much
social conditioning going on,' she says. 'This journey is about
digging into those foundations, examining them and finding out
how they've influenced your behaviour and your experience
through your whole life. The good news!! You can change all of
those foundations and start telling yourself different stories; it
will have a huge impact on your choices and experience and
help you decide what relationships in your life truly serve you.
As part of this work, which I call 'living beyond labels', you may
decide that labels you've been given or given yourself do express
your identity, or they may not be right for you and you'll find
other words or ways to describe, name and express that. Most
importantly you're being you!'

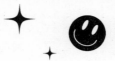

Yvonne's Story

Yvonne, 32, from Belfast, came out in 2018 and is a proud trans, non-binary autistic person.

Growing up, I went through countless cycles of starting new jobs or university courses and then dropping out, leaving or being fired. I always felt that I must not be applying myself enough, and couldn't understand why everyone else around me was managing to graduate and get amazing jobs. I felt stuck.

In 2018, I came out as non-binary and it felt like part of the puzzle clicked into place.

Then, at the start of the pandemic, my sister's friend was diagnosed with ADHD. I began to dig deep into both autism and ADHD and could really recognise myself in a lot of the accounts I read. I tried hard to get a diagnosis and received a referral, but then the clinic that referred me shut down. I've been trying to get a diagnosis for three years now and have had NHS licensed professionals tell me I should be able to get one, but with waiting lists so long, it feels impossible unless I go private.

Luckily, I'm confident with my self-diagnosis, but a clinical diagnosis would help me get the medication I need in order to concentrate.

Now I can identify fully as a trans, non-binary autistic person, I feel so much more confident in who I am. I think there's a higher rate of trans neurodivergent people because we consider things and think about them very intensely – we break away from what's expected of us. Looking back, I definitely repressed my stims and the way I self-soothe, as people told me they were 'weird'. But now I only mask when I'm with people I feel unsafe around, those who could judge me for my appearance or for being openly autistic. There are definitely people in my life who are resistant to or unsupportive of my diagnosis and current attempts at unmasking, but I've realised this is something I need to do for myself. A lifetime of masking has caused so much trauma; it's simply not worth it to keep doing it all the time! I have not had to remove anyone from my social group, but I'm prepared to do so if necessary.

Thankfully I have a lovely group of friends now. A lot of that was absolute luck, because of the journey I've been on and because of the sorts of people I gravitate towards. I think we often end up together by accident as our communication style and views tend to be quite similar or we've already been excluded by other groups. There is also a big crossover between the autistic and trans communities, and as I'm trans I've met quite a few more autistic/ADHD people through that community. I'm really happy to have found my people, who I can be myself around.

We could probably write a whole book on this stuff (and many people have), and there's no way we can fit into one chapter everything that encompasses sex and our sexual behaviour.

That stuff is so unique! We've just tried to outline our experiences as best as we can so as to open up the conversation around sex and, hopefully, make you feel able to explore your own self so much better.

Relationships

Is it any wonder that when we first begin to unpick what our diagnoses mean SO much comes up that it can feel overwhelming?! Your spicy brain doesn't define you, but it will impact almost every area of your life.

Lots of what we discussed in Chapter 11 on family and friends and in our discussions about sex comes into play here too, so check back in on the stories and advice from earlier. That said, our romantic relationships are unique: we spend the most amount of time with our partners, and for a healthy relationship to truly work, we need to show them exactly who we are and for them to accept that. That can be hard, particularly for women who have been taught to please their partner, no matter the cost to their own wellbeing (that shit is ingrained).

How your neurodivergence impacts your relationship will be totally different to how we've experienced it, but ultimately what we've learned is that self-acceptance is the key to joyful romantic relationships.

Mia on ... relationships

As I got older, I jumped from relationship to relationship. Even when I did slow down and get into longer-term relationships, I'd find other ways to make my life fast-paced: I'd throw myself into work, or create projects for myself, such as decorating my house again and again! Looking back, all of this was symptomatic of the fact that I couldn't relax, and being constantly on the go gave me a sense of control that masked the fact that I was avoiding processing my feelings. Being busy was a coping mechanism. Then, a relationship that I'd been in for five years broke down. It was a horrible break-up that coincided with a period of about eight months when I just couldn't get out of bed. I'd phone Jess crying, and a lot of friendships in my life broke down, too, because I had run out of energy and all the years of masking were catching up with me. Not long after, I had my ADHD and autism realisation, and I was forced into re-evaluating my needs. Constantly jumping between relationships and projects had been masking the fact that there was something going on for me that I hadn't yet addressed.

I'd also stayed in relationships for longer than I needed to, out of comfort, because being autistic means that the unknown can feel scary. When I met my current partner, it was the first time I'd entered into a relationship actually being my true, unmasked self.

Jess on ... relationships

We once designed a social media graphic of a stick figure surrounded by little bonfires. It was captioned: 'Lighting fires just to keep myself warm.' It summed up where I was at that time. I'm definitely a relationship person and I work hard at relationships. I want to be a good partner. A good friend. To know myself. I love hard and, as a result, I have some incredible people around me.

But in the past – pre-realisation, and as I worked to unmask – I would pick fights because I was bored. I was itchy in my own company and would then be like, 'Okay, am I going to seduce you or am I going to argue with you?' Like Mia using sex for stim-seeking, I was doing the same with arguments. I think both of us, as we've started to understand ourselves better, have also begun to recognise when under-stimulation is driving our behaviour.

I don't do things by halves. I either love something or I hate it. Everything is very intense. This has seen me completely immerse myself in relationships or people. I've been in four relationships, and they've all been fairly long-term. Some of those were with people who took advantage of how hard I love, and how hard I trust. I was cheated on and I was betrayed, and constantly let down. I took a lot of shit. I was vulnerable, people-pleasing and carrying around trauma. I was often in therapist mode, thinking I could fix people.

I'd like to tell you that I have an easy answer when it comes to escaping these (slightly destructive) patterns, but it largely comes down to me getting to know myself. And if it wasn't already clear, that's not a particularly comfortable process. I know how to meet my needs better than ever before, and it has drastically improved how I show up not only for myself, but also in my relationships.

I now consider how much energy I'm asking of my partner when I make requests essentially to be entertained. Now I'm better in tune with what I need to do to relax or wind down, I also see my partner meeting his own needs and relaxing differently. I want him to feel peaceful and balanced, just as I know I deserve now.

It's a healthy relationship with a very balanced amount of love and time spent together, one where I feel able to voice the rest of my needs (which hasn't always been the case in previous relationships). We've committed ourselves to being in a relationship that allows us both to thrive, and to feel safe, supported and heard. I think that's key. If your partner isn't willing to meet you where you need to be met, it can cause more shame on top of what you're already battling with, and that's clearly not what you need.

How to tear up the relationship rule book

It can be really hard to work out all of this huge stuff while also navigating a relationship with someone you love. As someone who works with a lot of different clients, relationship coach Natalie Roberts's advice below can be applied to absolutely everyone – whether you consider yourself neurotypical, neurodivergent, neuroqueer ... You do you. It can also be applied to many kinds of relationship, not just romantic ones. It's just super-applicable, brilliant advice ...

- ⚡ **It's going to be okay:** 'I've been doing this work for nearly 10 years and there's still a narrative out there that neurodiverse relationships (typically defined as any relationship that features neurodivergence or a mix of neuro-identities) inevitably don't work. That's a myth and actually really harmful. It's simply not a done deal that just because you're neurodivergent you're going to have unresolvable issues within your relationship. Yes, my work is focused on supporting neurodiverse relationships, so difference is absolutely a part of what's challenging and we need new ways to approach that. However, 80 per cent of what I'm typically addressing with clients is the effects of cumulative and persistent stress from not knowing about neurodiversity (for their whole lifetime or for years in a relationship) and unhealthy relationship dynamics that have them on a hamster wheel of unresolved issues. Being open to examining all of this helps you understand yourself more, recover from the stress of it all, and gives you new ways to be in and experience your relationships in a healthier way.'

- ⚡ **It begins with being open to exploring who you are:** 'Someone who realises they're neurodivergent may notice how often they're masking and want to discover who they are without that mask. Whilst the psychological burden of masking is typically much more for neurodivergent people, the truth is that to be loved, to be accepted or included, we all mask. This has a significant impact on all aspects of our health and wellbeing and beyond that in our relationships with others. So, when clients come to me – whether they're neurodivergent or neurotypical – with issues in their relationship, the first thing I say is, "Okay, let's redirect the attention for now away from your partner/the relationship and back to you." First, let's figure out "Who am I and how do I be me?" and from there it's about asking, "How can I be that version of me with you?" So often what happens is that we become another version of ourselves for the people we love. We need to learn how to be ourselves again.'

⚡ **Examine what you've been taught or learned:** 'We have been told so many stories about what a healthy, happy relationship and life should look like and who we should be and how we should be working to get that. I invite clients to think about what their stories and expectations of themselves, a partner and a relationship have been and then ask where have those come from; their culture, their childhood, or relationships in adulthood too? How are these stories and expectations working for them? When we're navigating difference, we need a different way to see and do all that other than what we've been presented with. It's about sidestepping and subverting mainstream culture and conditioning. It's embracing unconventional ideas and different ways to figure out who you actually are, what actually works for you and makes you happy on your own terms. Healthier ways of relating, that also support how different you are, change everything.'

⚡ **Consonance over compromise:** 'Compromise is touted as a common strategy within healthy relationships, and perhaps for some it works. But in a neurodiverse relationship, when you can be different and maybe opposites on many things, to compromise means both of you having to move a long way from who you are in order to find "middle ground". So you're living in the middle ground, and no one is happy there. You resent what you've given up; your partner resents what they've given up. A different strategy would be consonance – finding the circumstances and compatibility in which everyone is okay, where everyone's needs, preferences and limits are known and catered for. Take sitting down each night for dinner as a family or as a couple who live together: we are taught that an ideal family eats together and talks about their day. But that may not work if you have different sensory needs, food issues or differences, social preferences or anxieties, even different energies from your days. For so long my family forced itself to do this, but now we just let it go. This week, with my step-son visiting, we had four family meals in a week, which is a lot for us. We agreed that my son would come to one of them, as his social capacity would be too drained for four, and that my husband, who experiences sensory overload and social anxiety, didn't have to speak if he didn't want to. Essentially, it's about creating a space where everyone feels comfortable being themselves.'

⚡ **You don't have to get everything from one person:** 'Lots of people have a belief that to be "soul mates" with someone you have to have the same interests and the same capacity and enjoy situations in exactly the same way. This – in all relationships, but particularly neurodiverse ones – is rarely possible. I can have the exact same morning with my husband and we will view it and experience it in a totally different way. I've let go of the idea that because he doesn't experience or enjoy some things the way I do, that means we're not compatible. Even something as simple as trying new food and restaurants, that's something we've realised I love and he doesn't, so I find other people to go to these places with, or I try them out on my own. Together, we go to restaurants he's familiar with and sometimes, one that I've sussed out already! It's not about going without, it's about doing it differently.'

⚡ **You'll know when it's time to go:** 'If you're doing all this inner work and the person you're with isn't doing the same, you may reach a place where you think, "Is this over? Am I with the right person?" Or maybe even beginning this inner work feels scary – fear of the unknown, fear of what you'll discover, fear of upsetting or losing someone if you change. Our culture tends to fear the unknown and very few of us like uncertainty or have helpful, healthy or maybe even any ways to begin or to navigate it! If your relationship's been struggling, you were always going to reach this question of whether someone is right or wrong for you – maybe you've asked yourself that for ages already. Here's the different truth I found. After doing the work, you'll be able to approach it from a completely different place. This time, you're not asking the question when you are scared, angry or blaming them and yourself ... You're no longer in a fearful place that's driving thoughts of whether to stay or go. Instead, from a place of self-worth, self-respect and self-confidence, you're asking yourself, "Is this the relationship for me? Is it supporting me to become all of me?" Once you know and understand yourself more, once you're clearer about that and know what you want and need from this healthier, happier place of being you, it actually becomes a much easier question to answer.'

Relationships can lead to the most gorgeous experiences of our lives, making us feel so happy and connected and safe, but so can embracing being single and building a supportive community around you. We want you to know that it's all possible and we hope you find it, however you decide you want that area of your life to look.

CHAPTER 13

Health, Fitness and Nutrition

- ⚡ How to access healthcare
- ⚡ Basic hygiene and self-care
- ⚡ Food and nutrition
- ⚡ Disordered eating
- ⚡ Exercise

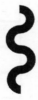

We both spent a long time feeling uncomfortable in our brains before deciding to take the unapologetic approach and embrace our neurodivergence. While we've spent a lot of time unpacking that in this book, in this chapter we'll be focusing on why so many of us feel uncomfortable in our bodies, too.

Basic self-care – by which we mean booking medical appointments, eating a balanced diet, exercising and maintaining hygiene, rather than bubble baths (although bubble baths are great) – is often hard to do when you have a brain like ours, partly because we can struggle to notice our body's cues. Narrow focus can create a tunnel-vision effect that limits awareness of the surrounding environment, while the attention differences commonly experienced by neurodivergent individuals can lead to difficulties in multitasking or processing multiple sensory inputs. This can make it difficult to notice physical cues indicating discomfort or fatigue.

As neurodivergent therapist Louise Taylor says, meeting our basic needs can be such a struggle. 'Everyone's experiences are so varied, and anxiety, past shame and trauma can all play into why we may find it hard to do something. Some people will find it hard to even know if they're hungry or thirsty, and others may find sensory difficulties with the feeling of water on the skin. At the heart of it all, everyone struggling to meet their basic needs should be treated with compassion.' Amen, Louise! Over time, as we've learnt how to work with our ADHD and autism, this stuff has become easier and we're a lot better at prioritising our health, fitness and nutritional needs than we've been in the past. Now, we're going to share what we've learnt.

Before we proceed, a disclaimer: as cis white women of a standard body shape, we're coming at this from a position of privilege. This stuff comes with a lot of stigma, because not showering or taking care of your appearance is so tied up with how society views a person and assesses their worth. If we begin to smell, or talk about how unhealthily we eat sometimes, we might get a bit of backlash, but we'd get nowhere near as much judgement as others with less privilege might face.

Accessing Basic Healthcare

The word 'health' has become such an umbrella term; it can be easy to forget that, at its root, it's about accessing the medicines and healthcare provisions we need. Many people have a real – and valid – fear of medical professionals and settings because they're from communities that have historically faced stigma and discrimination from these services, or even experienced it personally themselves. Layer the stigma of ADHD or autism on top of that, and it's not super-hard to understand why someone might feel apprehensive about accessing formal healthcare.

Neither of us can remember the last time we went to the dentist, and when it comes to registering with new doctors, we can take **months** to get round to it. There are varying reasons, for each of us, as to why we find meeting these basic healthcare needs so impossible – it can be as simple as sensory issues from brushing your teeth (**JESS:** I've recently switched to using a sensitive toothbrush and the sensory difference it's made has been wild), or anxiety around dealing with medical professionals and admin. If you feel the same, we see you. In Chapter 5, we talked about how the current healthcare system isn't really cut out for meeting the needs of neurodivergent people in terms of getting an ADHD or autism diagnosis, but it's also not equipped to help neurodivergent people when they want to use the service for health needs that are unrelated to their neurodivergence. Take getting a smear test, for example. They can be lifesaving, and posters everywhere remind us to book one without fear. That's great – and we should – but smear tests can be so much more uncomfortable for neurodivergent people because of our heightened sensory awareness. The same applies to getting injections, having a cannula inserted and having blood taken. A 2022 Care Quality Commission report found that in addition to the usual hesitation that people have when attending appointments like this, neurodivergent people can feel overwhelmed by the bustling medical environment and anxious as they don't know what to expect, and can find it difficult to convey to the professionals what they might need.[1] So, we don't go. Obviously, that's not a good idea. We shouldn't be putting off vital appointments, but sticking your head in the sand can sometimes feel the softest, safest option.

That said, over time, we've learnt how to make accessing healthcare easier on our ND brains. Here are our top tips:

- ⚡ **Use the NHS app:** You can re-order prescriptions and book appointments on it easily, without having to interact with anyone.

- ⚡ **Prepare yourself before appointments:** Ahead of time, give some consideration to how to make it easier for yourself. For example, we don't like going to new places and COVID-19 vaccinations were often in pop-up venues, so we'd call in advance and ask for parking advice and for information on exactly what would happen when we got there. If we didn't, we'd feel anxious about it all day. Let's be honest, these calls won't always be met with kindness, but get into the habit of doing what you need to make yourself feel better.

- ⚡ **Communicate your needs:** Explain the accommodations you need to doctors, doctors' receptionists and nurses. We say, 'I have an appointment with you and I have ADHD and autism. In order to make the experience manageable for me, could you dim the lights?' If we didn't take steps to manage our anxiety, we'd feel sick or become so frozen we wouldn't go. It's scary, but the more you ask for these accommodations, the more neurodivergent needs are taken into consideration, which means you'll be helping all the other ADHD and autism badasses who come after you.

Hygiene, Wellbeing and Self-Care

Although these things might sound 'soft', not feeling able to take care of yourself can impact your mental health. We feel ashamed for not showering every day, or not being able to stick to a 'skincare routine'. Women are often made to feel 'less than' if their appearance or personal hygiene doesn't meet with soci-etal standards of decorum and prettiness (and there's a whole world of patriarchal standards involved here that we're not going to go into). We now refuse to feel bad about ourselves. We're calling this state of mind **aggressive acceptance**, in that it **has** to be loud, brash and angry in order to break through all that other shit in our heads.

Jess on ... hygiene

I'm going to be real with you here. I find getting in the goddamn shower so taxing, and a lot of neurodivergent people feel the same. One of the things I find challenging is how many steps are involved. A task can feel so overwhelming that I ... just ... won't ... do ... it ... With showering, you have to find a towel, undress, turn the shower on, get under the water, wash yourself and then, even once you're out, you then have to GET DRY! GET DRESSED! DRY YOUR HAIR! By that point I've already done so many things it's like, um, where's my gold star?! All that energy used up and I'm **still** not done?! Now, I try to make the steps more fun, whether that's adjusting the environment so the lighting is nicer, or putting on a favourite song. Integrating elements of novelty is a way of helping ADHD brains to cope, so I'll add these fun tweaks to tasks that I find annoying. For example, I've switched to a coconut-flavour toothpaste, which means I actually enjoy brushing my teeth, and I put my towel on the radiator before a shower so it feels all cosy once I get out. They're simple things, but they make the experience **so** much nicer.

Mia on ... hygiene

I once didn't shower for so long that I developed a skin condition on my scalp (did I just share that with the world?). My hair would physically ache, it needed washing that badly. For me, it's less about the steps involved and more to do with the **sensation** of showering – of water on my skin, of having wet hair ... Honestly, I'm shuddering just thinking about it. I struggle with coordination, too, so drying and getting back into clothes ... ugh.

I've navigated all this by learning that I can take care of myself on my own terms. I don't need to do anything in a particular order; it doesn't matter if I shower first thing or I don't put on a body moisturiser afterwards. I celebrate that I've managed at all. I've also found that creating feel-good rituals makes such a difference to my wellbeing. They change week to week; sometimes it can be putting on a favourite outfit, but other times it's about running myself an indulgent bath. It has to make me feel good and it has to feel manageable. I've also invested in a decent hairdryer so that I don't need to have wet hair for too long.

Balancing fun and rest

We discussed in the previous chapter how some studies suggest that ADHD could be linked to low dopamine levels. Not enough is yet known to make this link concrete, but we do know that ADHDers need stimuli to focus on, so it stands to reason that finding balanced ways to stimulate your brain is key to enhancing your overall wellbeing. We've been trying to find ways to inject more 'healthy' fun into our lives (i.e. in a way that doesn't involve running out and grabbing a bottle of wine and the nearest person we can shag) for a while. The usual suspects – exercise, eating well, meditation, sleep and rest (more on those in a minute) – all apply, but here are some of the other things we've found that **really** work:

- ⚡ **Prioritise fun:** Our society puts a lot of value on productivity, but it's vital that we make time for the things that bring us joy. Note down the things that make you happy and do them more. Also, introduce new, fun things into your life – your ND brain craves novelty.
- ⚡ **Listen to music:** Several brain-imaging studies have found that listening to music increases activity in the reward and pleasure areas of the brain, which are rich with dopamine receptors.[2] Songs that make us feel something tend to have a better effect, so go with what you are feeling and sing it out loud.
- ⚡ **Get your glow on:** What makes you feel really good? You know the kind when you leave the house and are like, 'I am THE SHIT.' Doing your make-up? Wearing comfy clothes? Even going out in your PJs? Whatever it is, do it. Dress up excessively to get your Tesco meal deal for no other reason than it makes you feel good.
- ⚡ **Be creative with your rest:** Not getting enough rest decreases the availability of certain types of dopamine receptors.[3] With fewer receptors, dopamine doesn't have anywhere to attach to. Sleep and rest are, therefore, vital. Play around with what rest looks like for you: for some it can look like going to the beach, for others it's playing a fun game on the Nintendo Switch.

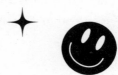

(Pssst … also remember, we live in a society that encourages us to 'chase' things for a dopamine hit, but regulation is the key word here – what goes up must come down. Pay attention to the things you are drawn to and question why. Take care of yourself.)

If you already like spending time on your own and you know how to do it in a healthy way, that's great. But if you don't, it's important to know how to spend time by yourself without falling into stim-seeking behaviours that you'd rather avoid.

Jess on … down time

I didn't know how to decompress in a way that was stimulating enough. I'd been sold this idea that relaxing was just sitting there with your own thoughts, like doing some deep breathing or journalling. That felt boring to me. I'd try and then end up pestering someone to spend time with me. But relaxation with stimulation does exist – Mia got really into crosswords for a while, and I love the colouring-in app Happy Color. I'd be like, 'I'm such an extrovert,' and think I **needed** other people to recharge, but actually I didn't know how to spend time by myself.

Whether it's making our poor brains work overtime to translate social cues or dealing with overwhelming social issues, we're often going at 1,000 miles an hour. Yet, when it's time to recover we are often so hard on ourselves (telling ourselves we're 'lazy' or punishing ourselves for seemingly not being able to cope as well as the others around us) and don't allow ourselves the rest we need. And did you know that, according to researcher Dr Saundra Dalton-Smith, there are SEVEN different types of rest?[5] Wild, right? She breaks them down as:

- ⚡ **Physical rest:** The classic, we suppose, where your body feels exhausted and craves the sofa. One of Dalton-Smith's tips is to 'choose to be still on purpose for five minutes', so setting a timer and just lying, as still as you can. Think the shavasana pose in yoga (that yummy bit where you just lie down at the end).
- ⚡ **Mental rest:** This is needed to stop your brain feeling as if it has 50 tabs open all at once. One recommended technique is to block out time for concentrating on just one task and putting your phone in another room so as not to feel the compulsion to respond to every message all the time.
- ⚡ **Emotional rest:** How much energy do you expend on worrying? It's one of the worst feelings in the world, and oh-so-natural to get caught in a worry or shame spiral. Take a break from it, Dalton Smith suggests, by writing everything down on paper and also identifying the people in your life who drain you and don't make you feel good, and distancing yourself from them.
- ⚡ **Social rest:** If you're someone who finds most social contact exhausting, you'll (hopefully) have got comfortable with making space in your life to be alone. But social rest doesn't just have to involve stretches of me-time. Instead, it's taking a rest from having to 'perform' or be someone you're not, so it can involve simply spending time with the people you feel you are your best and most sparkly self with.

- ⚡ **Sensory rest:** So many of us neurodivergent peeps suffer from sensory overload, with our brains and bodies having to work hard to process little irks, whether it's sounds or feelings. For sensory rest we need to pull ourselves into a safe, quiet place away from all of that, even for just a small amount of time.
- ⚡ **Creative rest:** Step. Away. From. Your. Emails. To find some creative rest we need to allow our brains to just **be**, away from the capitalist expectations placed on us. Basically, it's spending time focusing on little things that bring us joy, rather than the things we feel we **should** be doing.
- ⚡ **Spiritual rest:** You don't need to practise any sort of religion to find this. Instead, spiritual rest is all about a feeling of belonging and meaning. This could come from meditation, volunteering – really anything where you find your own peace.

So, how do we manage to get all that rest? It's tough, but begin by SAYING NO. And guess what? That might mean saying no to things we enjoy. Just because we get excited by an idea, that doesn't always mean it's a good idea.

Before you agree to something, remember:

- ⚡ Check in with your capacity (hello, unpredictable energy levels!).
- ⚡ You're allowed to find tiring things that other people don't.
- ⚡ You're allowed to ask questions before agreeing.
- ⚡ Not every opportunity needs to be taken, especially if it doesn't match your worth.

Sleep

We can't get no sleep. No, seriously, we can't. While trouble sleeping is an issue for a lot of people, studies have shown that neurodivergent people are more likely, from childhood, to suffer with sleep disorders such as insomnia.[4] But the real kicker is that we probably need more sleep and rest because of all the energy we're expending trying to fit into a neurotypical society.

These are the things that we've found help us get a better night's sleep:

- **Think about what happens before bed.** Are you scrolling and absorbing several other people's thoughts at the speed of light just before you rest your head on that pillow? Are you sat in a bright room, desperately trying to find anything to keep you entertained? If yes, it's probably not helping. We love reading long-form content, using mood lighting – or dimming the lights – and using colouring-in apps instead.
- **Be honest about your caffeine intake.** If you consume caffeine in any form, how late into the day are you having it? We both drink coffee either as a way to avoid doing what we're doing or to break up the day, but try not to drink it too late in the day (said with zero judgment, of course).
- **Try supplements.** Don't go taking any supplements before checking with your doctor (snore, we know, but it'd be irresponsible of us to exclude that disclaimer) but

we've found there are a couple that really help with our sleep, like magnesium and CBD. Both *have* actually made a noticeable difference for us.

Food and Nutrition

Please be aware that in this section, we'll be talking a bit about our own experiences with eating. **Trigger warning:** Parts of our stories contain mentions of disordered eating. If that's something you're struggling with right now, you may want to skip past this bit. We've chosen to share it as we really want you to know how having a brain like ours can disrupt your relationship with food, and that if it's affecting you too, you're not alone.

Being neurodivergent can really influence your relationship with food (as can, you know, society), because a lot of the traits associated with ADHD and autism might impact your eating habits as well. Anne Pemberton, a functional medicine and nutrigenomics practitioner, mum of an autistic child, and speaker for Food for the Brain (a charity dedicated to generating awareness about the importance of nutrition and lifestyle for mental well-being and cognitive health) says that neurodivergent brains might exhibit the following traits when it comes to eating:

- ⚡ A lack of interest in food.
- ⚡ Struggling to process all the different steps in a recipe.
- ⚡ Being far too tired to cook due to autistic burnout.
- ⚡ Feelings of unworthiness after years of trauma (you might feel unworthy of nourishing yourself).

- ⚡ Sensory sound issues, including noise from extractor fans and blenders in kitchens.
- ⚡ Sensory texture issues, such as a dislike of certain textures limiting food choices.
- ⚡ Sensory smell and taste issues – the sense of smell can either be heightened or non-existent, while your sense of taste can be heightened or diminished. With diminished taste and smell there is less motivation to eat.
- ⚡ Some people relate food to negative situations, such as being in a noisy cafeteria at school, which creates food trauma.
- ⚡ High levels of anxiety around many daily activities, such as cooking and eating.

That's A LOT to contend with! So remember, please be gentle with yourself and know that if you are struggling with food, as Jess talks about in the pages that follow, it's not your fault.

ADHD, Autism and Nutrition

Some studies have linked ADHD and autism with certain nutritional deficiencies and suggested that supplementing the diet might have benefits.[6] Nutrients we often lack include omega-3 fatty acids, zinc and magnesium. Speak to your doctor if you're concerned and want to learn more about how this might be affecting you.

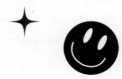

Neurodivergent Brains and Disordered Eating

Given how predisposed our brains are to struggling with food and eating, it's not surprising that research shows that being neurodivergent and eating disorders/disordered eating are closely linked. According to the eating disorders charity Beat,[7] between 4 per cent and 23 per cent of people with an eating disorder are also autistic.[8] One study suggests that the risk of people with ADHD developing an eating disorder (ED) is three-fold compared to those without ADHD,[9] with women and girls possibly being more at risk than men and boys,[10] in part due to going undiagnosed with ADHD more often. Another review of 16 studies found a prevalence rate of ADHD in people with eating disorders ranging from 1.6 per cent to 18 per cent.[11] In comparison, the prevalence of ADHD in the general population is about 2.5 per cent.

Jess on … her relationship with food

For as long as I can remember, my relationship with food has been complicated. Growing up in the noughties, I was surrounded by toxic messages from the media, and it all sank in. I can remember being at school and testing myself to see how long I could go without eating. Friends warned me that my behaviours weren't healthy, but I didn't listen. I've felt out of control for so much of my life (and I didn't always know that it was because of my autism and ADHD), but controlling my food intake was one way that I could feel as though I was in the driving seat. At university, I'd go through phases of not eating much, binge eating and having in my head lists of foods that were 'safe' to eat. I didn't know it then, but this is a sign of avoidant restrictive food intake disorder (ARFID), where you have highly selective eating habits and avoid certain foods (see page 277). I was obsessed by calorie counting and weighing myself.

Being diagnosed with lupus in my third year made me rethink my entire relationship with, well, pretty much everything, including food. I realised that always eating the same three meals (pesto on pasta, beans on toast and ... cereal) probably wasn't going to be the route to helping my body thrive or reduce my inflammation. Ditto my addiction to Pepsi Max, pink Lucozade and Fanta Lemon. I cut out alcohol entirely (booze made the symptoms flare up like a bitch) and added as many fruits and vegetables to my diet as I could manage.

I was treating my body better than I ever had, but I also began to notice that the weight was dropping off me. I began to get addicted to stepping on the bathroom scales, watching the number go down. I hadn't started eating this way to lose weight – it was for my health – but it quickly became toxic. Looking back, again it was a need for control. By this point, Mia had moved away; I missed her so much and my lupus also meant I was experiencing a lot of pain and swelling, which was all tied in with adjusting to living with a lifelong condition. In short, it was a total clusterfuck.

Looking back at pictures of that time, I feel so sad for that girl. At the time, I found it really hard to see a way out, but bit by bit, things got easier. When I figured out first that I was an ADHDer and then that I was autistic five years after uni, it helped because I was able to see that so many traits can be connected to food and eating patterns. I can recognise that, because of the ADHD, the steps in cooking are hard for me, as is waiting for things to be ready, but with my autism it's a texture and taste thing.

Jess's Food Hacks:

⚡ **Make piña colada smoothies:** I got myself a cheap blender and always have fruit in the freezer. I'll chuck it into the blender, whizz it up with some milk and then put it in a wine glass so it feels like a bouji cocktail.

⚡ **Find snacks you love:** I know now that there are certain things I really like and I rely on them. For example, protein bars – there are a few flavours of one brand that I get again and again. They're good to have in the house to grab if I feel hungry.

⚡ **Minimise prep:** I've memorised a few meals that involve simply putting a mix of ingredients into the oven (or my air fryer) with very little food prep. It means I'm spending less brain energy on thinking about mealtimes.

I now haven't weighed myself in years. I concentrate on putting good things in my body and I'm not too hard on myself. A big part of it has been to let go of any shame. Do I need to order a takeaway because it's too much to think about cooking? Do it! Am I going to have cereal for dinner? Yes! I try to be kind to myself and realistic as to what I can achieve, but I still struggle and think I always will. If someone is around me talking about weight-loss I have to say, 'I'm pleased you're feeling happy, but I find that hard to hear,' as it's a slippery slope. I think it's okay to accept that I'll always find this stuff hard, while appreciating how far that I have come.

You're Not Alone ...

Seriously. The more we talk about our experiences, the more we realise how many others have gone through something similar.

There are a multitude of reasons why us ND folk are more likely to suffer from disordered eating, or formal eating disorders, Eleanor Speakman – one of Beat's senior helpline advisors – tells us. 'Eating disorders are caused by a multitude of factors: genetic, biological and social triggers ... and these can often be experienced differently in neurodivergent people, although research into this is currently limited.' Controlling food intake can be a way of managing difficult emotions and providing a sense of control, she adds. 'There can be a lot of high-level anxiety [around eating], which can lead to a rule-driven behaviour [that] develops because of the difficulties that someone may experience in everyday life. For someone with ADHD there could also be impulse-control issues, and behaviours towards food may be an attempt to emotionally regulate or seek stimulation.'

Research suggests that avoidant restrictive food intake disorder (ARFID) is one of the most common eating disorders among neurodivergent people, Eleanor explains. 'This is when someone avoids certain foods, limits how much they eat or does both, but beliefs around weight or body shape are not the reasons why. Instead, it's down to sensory issues, such as a negative feel around the smell, taste or texture of certain foods. Some people even strongly dislike the feeling of food in their stomach. There may also be concerns about the consequences of eating or a low interest in eating. ARFID can look quite different from one person to another.'

It's important for us to remember, she stresses, that although they may have physical indicators, eating disorders are a mental illness. 'To really recognise if you're struggling, or someone you know is struggling, consider the thoughts and feelings around eating, and how much it's impacting your daily life. If [you are] having concerns about eating and notice a change in behaviour and thinking to do with that, it could indicate a problem. Food should not cause emotional distress.'

If you remember one thing, says Eleanor, it should be that you should reach out as soon as possible: 'We would always recommend speaking to a loved one in the first instance. But if you don't want to do that, Beat also has a helpline. Your GP would also be a step, but we know that can be really difficult for neurodivergent people, and so we recommend things like making notes of your feelings before seeing a medical professional. We know that can be really difficult for neurodivergent people, and we recommend things like making notes of your feelings beforehand, asking if you can bring a friend or family member to the appointment and asking for the GP to make adjustments, such as turning down the light, to help with any sensory difficulties.'

Nikki's Story

Nikki, 31, from Hereford, has ADHD and works on an eating disorder ward for teens. She's also suffered with disordered eating herself.

The majority of the patients we see are anorexic or have ARFID. Often for people with neurodivergent brains eating isn't necessarily a priority. Autistic people might get stuck in hyperfocus and spend a day without eating, and then easily fall into a restrict-and-binge cycle. Or, often due to sensory issues, autistic people really narrow their diet down and they can only eat the same things over and over again. That could then become an issue, as more of an ARFID presentation. It's so complicated as there's no clear-cut answer.

It can also be difficult to separate what's someone's ADHD and autism and what's an eating disorder. I think for anybody who is constantly thinking about food and how they look, and are very strictly avoiding foods or becoming obsessive about them or exercise, should reach out for some help. Our aim with all our young people is that they have both a variety of food to be healthy in the physical sense, with vitamins and nutrients, but also that they can enjoy food – having Friday-night pizza and birthday cakes.

Looking back, my undiagnosed ADHD definitely impacted my own eating habits. I went through a period of time when I wasn't eating, but I was also purging up my food. I think now it was an attempt to stimulate my brain, that there was an element of getting a dopamine hit, in seeing how long I could go without eating. My job has definitely helped me manage that, as has my diagnosis and being on ADHD medication. I have real empathy for what my patients are going through, and how hard it is for them. But I also see how often we do manage to help people find another way and to get to that healthy place with their eating again.

Isn't it funny (not funny ha-ha, more we **have** to laugh or we'll cry) how so many of the things that we're told in life are simple are anything but? Cooking and maintaining a healthy diet is one of them. We know it's not just our community who are patronised either: lower-income households are continually chastised for struggling with 'maintaining a healthy diet' by people with no understanding of their circumstances. If you're struggling, please don't punish yourself for it, but also, vitally, if you're really worried about your eating habits, you don't need to deal with it alone, so do speak to someone.

Exercise

Moving our bodies is a sure-fire way to feel better – that's not exactly ground-breaking information, but it's not always easy to achieve when you have an ND brain. There's a lot of toxic messaging out there around exercising – you know the type: 'No excuses!' 'Get up, get out!' 'But **we're not lazy**!' we want to scream. We're not exercising regularly because we're mentally and physically exhausted by the expectations placed on us every single day.

Of course, there are plenty of autistic and ADHD people who are bloody brilliant at exercise, but if you're not someone who intuitively loves working out, we wanted to show you that you're not alone, because the reality is that being a neurodivergent badass does add some barriers. 'The fitness industry is really behind when it comes to making exercise accessible for everyone,' explains Dale Robertson, who set up (and we think this is so awesome) Scotland's first ever gym for disabled people, DR Inclusive Fitness & Wellbeing, where he trains neurodivergent clients of all ages. 'I used to train in a space that was seemingly accessible, as it was on the ground floor and had wheelchair accessibility. But there were still social and communication barriers for disability that were perhaps more prevalent than access issues.' These can include (for neurodivergent people in particular) sensory issues (such as weights slamming/noise pollution from classes) and difficulties in reading social cues (gym etiquette is a whole other form of etiquette). Then there are motor difficulties, which could stop some of us from doing certain required movements in sports.

The truth is that what constitutes a barrier to exercise is incredibly varied, dependent on who you are and what your life has been like so far. 'It's amazing what a difference small adaptations can make,' Dale explains. 'One client of mine, an autistic woman, likes to know what we're going to be doing in advance, so there's no surprises. Another needs me to break down each step of the move for her, each time. We also have gym equipment with different handles that for some people can reduce

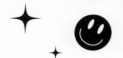

sensory issues. It's a very tailored approach, examining the barriers and seeing what changes can be made to ensure exercise is enjoyable.'

We wish there could be a Dale Robertson gym on **every** corner, but unfortunately he's only got one in Edinburgh. So how can someone enjoy exercise without the support of trainers like him? In the following pages, we've outlined our own journeys, but Dale encourages examining your own barriers and history when it comes to fitness. 'It can be really common to have a bad experience and then associate exercise with that bad experience from then on,' he says. 'Particularly as so much of our introduction to exercise can be PE lessons in school – environments that are often not set up in an accessible way at all. Even the nature of how some PE teachers (and trainers) speak could be a barrier, as an autism trait could be struggling to follow direct instruction. A lot of fitness language is inaccessible in itself.' Erm, could that be any more true?

Once you've identified what your barriers might be, you could find ways to work around them (but don't ever feel you have to, remember bestie, these barriers aren't on you to change), Dale advises. 'So, if you struggle with a busy gym environment, try to go at quieter times, or look up the class timetable online and avoid going when there's a class on, as that can cause noise pollution.' He also recommends looking into what motivates you to exercise. 'One of my clients is not in any way motivated by weight-loss goals, so instead we set performance-based goals. Another, who is a power lifter, cannot lift the weight if she knows how heavy it is, so we don't tell her.'

All this, we're very aware, doesn't just rely on having a Dale Robertson gym round the corner, but also having an adequate disposable income to join a gym or hire a personal trainer, which many of us don't have due to high rates of unemployment in our community. Time can also be such an issue, as well as unpicking old trauma from bad gym experiences. We don't want you to feel as if we're lecturing you in any way, as it can be so hard to escape negative thoughts such as, 'When have I ever stuck to anything in my entire life?' and 'I'm just a let-down; I'll never manage.' It's only recently, as our confidence has built up, that we've been able to even consider adding exercise to our lives, and this is what we've learnt ...

What works for Jess

- ⚡ **Find your motivation:** People with ADHD are motivated by interest, novelty and fun. Personally, I get so bored of things that aren't stimulating enough, so I'll look on YouTube for fun, varied classes.
- ⚡ **Watch out for weight-loss messaging:** This could be really triggering for me, so I have to be careful. The Yeh Yoga Company classes make a powerful point by never mentioning it, while MissFits Workout offers online dance workouts for people who might not feel comfortable in a gym environment.
- ⚡ **Find a walking buddy:** Mia and I started to take walks while talking on the phone. We're not physically together, but I still find it helpful to have someone to walk 'with'.
- ⚡ **Romanticise it:** I make working out more appealing to my brain by adding in novelty elements, like taking a nice water bottle to a class or wearing fun activewear.

What works for Mia

- ⚡ **Find a quiet space:** I'm very all or nothing and there was a long period of my life where I did go to the gym quite frequently. I'd managed to find a small hotel gym near where I lived, and I'd go on the treadmill and then go for a swim. It worked well because I find bigger gyms way too loud and overstimulating.

- ⚡ **Challenge yourself (but don't take it too far):** Sometimes, my brain seems to want me to be in competition with myself (as we've talked about, 'stim-seeking' behaviours like this are common in ND brains). Whenever I went to the gym I'd track calories as a motivator, and it can make me feel that if I'm not smashing a goal then what's the point? But that's not necessarily healthy. Now, I try to motivate myself to do gentler forms of exercise, such as swimming.

- ⚡ **Know what feels good for you:** What feels good for my mind and body has a huge influence on how I exercise. I now seek out things that don't entail dealing with sensory sensitivities, for example. I also know that having ADHD means that my brain in the morning can often feel like it's full of bees, so going for a walk before I start work can help me feel more grounded. Being ND means that towards the end of the day I can get easily overstimulated and find it hard to switch off, so that's where swimming or perhaps doing some gentle yoga can calm things down, to make sure I don't carry the stress of my day into the evening.

Ironically, as soon as we changed the goal from 'being better' to 'being gentler and realistic' when it came to self-care, we seemed to manage more than we did previously. We're realising that there are plenty of hacks and alternative ways of doing things that make it feel a little easier (or less boring, to be real with you), and that there are some days when we'll manage it no problem.

But you know what? We also now care a lot less. Do we have dirty hair more often? Maybe! Do we have an irregular shower-ing routine? Uh, yeah. But are we celebrating what we manage, and refraining from intertwining our struggles with our 'worth' as humans? Also yes. Ultimately, we're no longer expecting ourselves to be able to manage it all. We're loosening our stand-ards, acknowledging what's difficult and leaning into what we DO feel good about. And we think you deserve the same.

> If you're worried about your own or someone else's health, you can contact Beat, the UK's eating disorder charity, 365 days a year on 0808 801 0677 (England only) or via their website: beateatingdisorders.org.uk

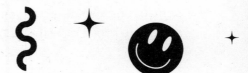

CHAPTER 14

Life Admin

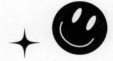

⚡ **Executive dysfunction and life admin**

⚡ **Facing necessary tasks**

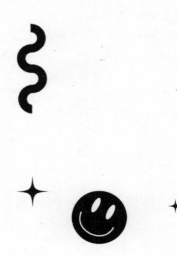

Take a look at our feed and it could easily look like we've got it all together. We often worry that our community think we're managing way better than we actually are; behind the curated posts, we're often really, really struggling to keep up with every ball that modern life demands we juggle.

In the past couple of months, we've:

- had to transfer the final £3 in our savings account to pay for antidepressants
- come off video calls so exhausted that we had to sleep all afternoon
- found ourselves overwhelmed by having to pay our phone bill on time.

The point is: this shit is hard. For people with ADHD and autism, keeping up with life admin is difficult for many reasons, one being that many of us have an aversion to being told what to do. Our brains also struggle with boring tasks. Successfully completing lots of life admin also heavily relies on our executive functions (those cognitive skills such as task prioritisation and time management that we discussed in Chapter 3). You might remember that executive **dys**function is a key signal of ADHD.[1] While there are some expectations we can let go of (no, we don't need a super-tidy house, thank you), there are some tasks that can't be skipped. After all, if we skip paying our bills, the consequences are real.

What Does Executive Dysfunction Look Like?

We talked about executive dysfunction in Chapter 3, but it comes into play in a big way when it comes to life admin. It's infuriating to know exactly what it is you need to get done, but to struggle to motivate yourself to do it. This is executive dysfunction and it's something that happens in our brains that makes the ordering of tasks and making decisions all the trickier. Some people don't like labelling it as ND behaviour – they feel it pathologises our lives – whereas we kind of like having a label for something we struggle with.

Being neurodivergent also impacts how we perceive time. If, like us, you find that your lack of perception of time has you floating through life not **really** knowing what day it is but throwing some charm around and somehow managing to make it work, this could be why. Neurodivergents can struggle with temporal processing abilities, which affect executing functioning. This interferes with our ability to perceive time accurately.

Here are some ways executive dysfunction shows up in our lives:

- ⚡ Walking past suitcases knowing we need to unpack them – yet not doing it.
- ⚡ Letting laundry sit in the basket for two weeks, which needs putting away, and knowing that until we do that we can't do more washing as the basket is full.
- ⚡ Not being able to close cupboard doors and drawers.

- ⚡ Having bags of clothes waiting to go to the charity shop for months.
- ⚡ Having piles of packages that need to be sent and only finding the energy to send them when the post office is closed.
- ⚡ Becoming so focused on something that we forget to take care of ourselves.

There's a lot of advice out there on how to deal with executive dysfunction – how to hack it to make it work for you – but a lot of it centres on you trying to adapt to a neurotypical way of being. If you want to investigate this, go on! But for us, it's about accepting that this is a part of us and trying our best to let go of societal expectations.

Five things to remember if you struggle with executive dysfunction

- ⚡ Forgetting things isn't a character flaw, whether your brain tells you that or not.
- ⚡ It doesn't have to be perfect! **Sometimes done is better than not at all** – give yourself permission to do a less-than-perfect job, bestie.
- ⚡ Don't let shame around being 'lazy' stop you from resting; shame is a totally useless concept anyway.
- ⚡ The neurotypical way isn't the only way.
- ⚡ The people around you don't need to understand your struggle for it to be real.

The ADHD/Autism Tax

Ever forgotten to return a library book and received a fine? Had to pay late fees on your bills? Had your mobile phone cut off because even though you had the money you didn't pay your bill? That's what we're talking about. So many people with ADHD and autism end up in dire straits with their finances because we go into freeze mode or find the steps for paying a bill too much. That, in turn, means we are often dealing with things at the last minute, which triggers fight-or-flight mode in us. And guess what? When we're in that trauma-response state, life feels so much harder. We just want you to know that we recognise that vicious circle. We know that a lot of what you're experiencing is down to past trauma, so please don't feel bad about yourself for getting trapped within it. It does get easier; the more you sit with that trauma and accept it, the stronger you will feel and the more equipped you will be to deal with it. If you are struggling with debt, contact a debt advice charity like Stepchange (www.stepchange.org).

Hey, You! You're Doing Okay

There are so many little life admin-y things etched into our society that, if you forget to do them, it can make you feel as if you're not a good person or that you're not a caring person. We're talking birthday cards, thank-you cards, sending messages of congratulation to people. It's so easy to let it affect your confidence when you miss these things ... You might end up just ignoring your phone or thinking, 'Well, shit, I forgot to send that card, so they hate me now,' and then just ... never ... getting ... in ... touch ... again. We've been in that spiral so many times. Just recently we had to message a friend to congratulate them for something and we forgot, but instead of beating ourselves up about it, we said to ourselves, 'It's okay, we've had a hard year. Life has been more difficult than usual to manage. This doesn't make us bad people.' Then we messaged simply saying, 'We just want you to know that even when we're quiet, we still really care about you and have been thinking of you.' Forgetting these things doesn't make you thoughtless or any less of a friend or partner. We all wish we had extra energy, but we don't. That's okay. We've attached so much moral value to things that don't really matter, such as outward appearances and keeping a tidy house. Let go of those expectations – your spicy brain will thank you for it.

But What About Those Tasks You Actually Do Need to Do?

A confession: we can't give you magic ways to make needing to book an appointment you've been putting off and then finding that you have to call back another time less draining, but we can suggest things that have worked for us, starting with getting in the zone. 'When I get in the zone I can accomplish anything' – sound familiar? Well, friends, that zone is your interest-based nervous system when it's fully engaged.

If you've never heard of this concept before, let us introduce you to Dr William Dodson, an ADHD expert, who found when working with clients that they were fully capable of motivation and paying attention, but struggled when trying to fit into productivity expectations placed on them by neurotypical people.[2] The thing is, neurotypical people have what is known as an 'importance-based nervous system', and that means that what motivates them to get tasks done is the outcomes, rewards and consequences (i.e. if I don't pay this bill, I will be fined).

However, people with ADHD have an interest-based nervous system, where what motivates us is interest, competition, novelty and urgency. Sometimes when you try to explain this to a person who doesn't understand, they'll say, 'You think I like paying bills? I don't like it. I do it because I have to.' That's entirely the point! They can recognise the consequences a lot more easily than people with our kind of nervous system. Interesting tasks for us will almost always take precedence, even when we know we'll be in serious trouble if we don't do it.

This is why a lot of us struggle with life admin jobs – because we are under-stimulated and bored by them. However, we can play a game with our brain by recognising that our interest-based nervous system is broken down into four main conditions and that one of these may be more motivating than the others. The key is to work out which works best for you. For example, when cleaning the kitchen could you:

- ⚡ treat yourself to a new scented cleaner? Put on some music? (Introducing novelty)
- ⚡ research some new cleaning hacks? (Providing interest)

⚡ invite friends over so you have to clean before their arrival? (Creating urgency)

⚡ set a timer and challenge yourself? (Competing)

And when you can't get in the zone? Here are some other things that have helped us navigate the seemingly endless reams of life admin we're faced with:

⚡ **Rant about it:** We've found speaking to someone who really doesn't care about said task, who has no emotional attachment to it at all, really helps. It might be boring AF for them to listen to, but they can usually remove the baggage from it and help you see it more clearly.

⚡ **Identify what's difficult about the situation:** Instead of saying, 'It's just fucking hard, I can't,' and leaving it at that (though we hear you; it is hard), try to examine **why** it's hard. Then see if there's another way to do that task. Because the world is designed for neurotypical people, we often think their way to approach tasks is the right way, even if we struggle with it. Besties, that's not the case! Figure out your own way.

⚡ **Stop shaming yourself:** No, you're not an awful human for not doing it in time, but guess what? Telling yourself you are drains you of energy, which then makes doing said task even harder. Being kinder to yourself will make things easier, we promise.

⚡ **Body doubling:** A funny thing we discovered is that there were some tasks we could only do if someone else was with us – this is known as body doubling. Grab a pal or video call them, with the intention of the pair of you doing the tasks you keep putting off together, whether that's tidying your room or replying to emails. Just having another person present keeps you grounded and focused on the task. It's like magic; if you encounter an obstacle, you can say it aloud and find a solution together, and that stops you spiralling into defeat. We experience quite intense, emotional reactions when things don't go according to plan, and if you've got someone keeping you on track when you're doing things, you're less likely to completely freak out.

⚡ **Lean on others:** When we talk about community, we really fucking mean it. I think when most people hear that word they think of community halls or swimming pools, but we mean breaking away from the hyper-independence our culture demands of us. There are so many places in the world that aren't like this, that work as a group and get shit done that way. That's what we mean – there's no shame in lacking skill in certain areas and leaning on a pal to help you out, whether that's body doubling (see above) or having your partner/flatmate pick up some tasks that you can't. We all have something to offer and can help each other out.

⚡ **Leave visual reminders:** Out of sight, literally out of mind, right? We forget so many things because of this, so now we just leave shit out so we can see it. Our partners will be like, 'Why was that bottle on the worktop?' and we'll be like, 'Doh, to remind us to clean something!'

⚡ **Task swapping:** This is sharing the smaller tasks within a task with someone else until it's completed, e.g. if you struggle with getting the laundry done, you might have an agreement that you load the washing into the machine and your housemate/partner puts it out to dry.

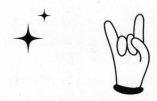

CHAPTER 15

Parenting

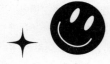

- ⚡ **Kirsti's story**
- ⚡ **Parenting a neurodivergent child**
- ⚡ **Getting a diagnosis for your child**

Besties with kids, we see you and you're doing great! But, as we're not parents ourselves, we wanted to hand this chapter over to Kirsti Hadley, founder of Generation Alphabet, an online space that creates a community of people who want to learn about and celebrate neurodiversity. She's someone we met through Instagram and who we adore. We literally say to each other all the time, 'Can Kirsti be our mum, too?' as the way she's parenting her child, Sonny (who uses they/them pronouns), is truly revolutionary. Kirsti uses any opportunity to speak up about what it's like to be a neurodivergent parent (she was diagnosed with ADHD and autism when she was 48) to a neurodivergent child (Sonny was diagnosed as autistic when they were nine). She's passionate that we should be changing the world, not the kids. That **if a child is struggling in school, it's not their fault; it's the system that isn't right for them**.

When we think back to our own childhoods – to the struggles we had at school, and how our parents tried their best but didn't have the language to speak to us or equip us for this world – we just wish there had been someone like Kirsti around to help guide the way.

Kirsti's incredible wisdom

'Mummy, when there's been so many doctors around ... why am I not fixed yet?' When my child, Sonny, said this to me one night in the bath, it was like a dagger in my heart. They're autistic and all the advice I'd been given by professionals up until that point had been, 'Don't tell them, just tell them they're different – say it's like we're in a fruit bowl and there's a banana, an apple and a pear ...' I had always thought it was a nice analogy, but it had felt wrong to me, as if we were gaslighting children when they tried to open up about how they feel.

That night I decided that, from then on, I was going to trust my gut and do what I thought was best for my child, not what I'd been told was best for my child. I turned to Sonny and I said, 'You are not broken, there's nothing wrong with you and you do not need to be fixed. That's not why there's been so many doctors. There are two types of brains: a neurodivergent brain and a neurotypical brain. Neither one is less than the other, they're just very different. And depending on which one you've got, it will dictate how you feel emotions, how you learn ...'

They listened quietly and then just turned around and said, 'Oh, cool.'

In lots of ways, Sonny seemed just like me. But in 2018, when they were six, they began hand-flapping and I thought I should investigate why. From then on I began the process of reading as much as I could and fighting for a diagnosis for Sonny. I didn't take any time to consider how what I was learning could apply to my own life, my own traits.

Then, in 2020, in quick succession my friend died from suicide, my mum died and then we went into lockdown. I was juggling so much and dropping so many balls, but I wasn't equipped to be able to say, 'This is why I can't cope.' I had a total mental break-down. Sonny was having daily meltdowns, I was having daily meltdowns, Sonny's dad left ... I felt like I was playing a game of Whac-a-Mole and every time I tried to get myself up, something would whack me down again. Until, eventually, I couldn't get up anymore.

I was diagnosed with PTSD first, in 2021, from the impact of that year but also from incidences in my childhood. It was during talking therapy for the PTSD that the psychologist suggested that, while pursuing a diagnosis for Sonny, I should perhaps consider one for myself.

The biggest change has been the ability to identify what my traits are and empowering Sonny to do the same. I can divide up my traits into my ADHD bits, my autistic bits and the bits that are based on what has happened to me throughout my life. That helps me understand which ones I can work on, and which ones I'm never going to be able to change. The parts I can't change I no longer apologise for, but I will communicate them. Neurodivergent people, and women in particular, carry a lot of guilt. Now my life is about fewer apologies, more explanations.

The brilliant thing about Sonny and me going through a diagno-sis at the same time is that we're having these conversations all the time, about what works for us and what doesn't, as there is lots of common ground and many similarities. Our personalities are also within that, though. We're different people, and we don't assume things. Before they go to sleep, Sonny likes to have a hair-dryer in one hand and a speaker playing Audible in the other. They like the soft, warm air and the white noise. One night, it was almost time for bed, so I asked them to switch the hair-dryer off, saying it was time to wind down. They didn't, so I told them again. That's when they said, 'You've told me twice now, so I can't do it.' Sonny, like I am, is really demand avoidant – they find it hard to comply with requests and aren't able to do certain things at certain times. Typical parenting would frame that moment as my child being disobedient. But instead, we came up with a solution together. I simply said, 'Oh, of course. Well, what are we going to do about that?' Sonny then asked if they could blow-dry themselves for two minutes, then I'd blow-dry them for two minutes, then I'd give the hair-dryer back as 'they had to switch it off themselves'. It worked.

After a meltdown, when everyone has calmed down, we'll talk about what triggered it and how I can help them. I don't position it as me 'teaching' Sonny, more like us discussing our needs together.

There is very little support out there for neurodivergent families, particularly within the school setting. If I had my way, I'd tear down the educational system and rebuild it from the ground up. We're seeing high levels of autistic children missing school,[1] and, currently, I home-school Sonny. I believe kids are dropping out of school because they're reaching burnout inside a system that isn't right for them. In an ideal world I'd want to see a mental-health-first approach to learning, rather than an academic approach. I always say to Sonny, 'Your self-esteem matters more than your grades.' Currently they're in equine therapy, where they're learning all about horses, and they love it! They say they hate learning, but it's clear they don't; they just hate the way traditional learning is set up.

Neurotypical society has always dictated how we live our lives, and what we have to do as parents to neurodivergent kids is unlearn what we've learnt and find our own ways to parent. That takes time, but it's also a rewarding journey. If we can teach our children to be their true selves from as early on as possible, then they are going to have fewer mental health problems, fewer hang-ups, and they'll be more accepting of others. Everyone should be able to learn how their brain works, and what's best for them.

Kirsti's Advice for Parents ...

- ⚡ **Neurodiversity is nothing to be scared of:** I still see a lot of resistance from parents about getting a diagnosis, particularly with autism. People think, 'I don't want an autistic child,' but I'm saying that you do. This is something to celebrate! Your child has the opportunity to get to know themselves from an early age, and that's wonderful.
- ⚡ **Relinquish power:** Take your time and treat your child as an equal. Really listen to them and how they choose to communicate with you.
- ⚡ **There is no such thing as bad behaviour:** Every type of behaviour is a method of communication, so be careful with your language. Don't use words like 'disruptive' or 'disobedient' – it will only reinforce how they feel about themselves. Make it about positive reinforcement, rather than negative statements.
- ⚡ **Give them power:** Particularly if there's a demand avoidance pattern of behaviour. It helps to ask them what they want and to ask them to do something, rather than telling them what to do.

⚡ **Lead by example:** I am not a perfect parent. I do lose my shit. When I do, I will own it and go back to Sonny and say, 'Mummy made a mistake there,' and then we discuss how things could go better next time.

⚡ **Prioritise self-care:** I didn't reach my own diagnosis until after I reached a complete mental breakdown and I was suicidal. No one should have to reach that point. I don't ever like to describe neurodivergent kids as challenging; instead, I say that, as parents, we are presented with challenging situations. That means you have to take care of yourself when you can. Take a bath, go for a walk, do a meditation. It really helps.

⚡ **Separate emotions from being:** I always say to Sonny that there are no bad feelings. I try to separate their own feelings from who they are. Of course, meltdowns are exhausting and upsetting, I'll admit that. I'll say, 'That was really exhausting for you, but that doesn't mean you're a bad person. It's a part of who you are.'

⚡ **Name things:** I call Sonny's meltdowns their 'angry'. But it also helps to ask your kids to identify and name their feelings themselves. It encourages them be more self-aware of their traits, which, in turn, helps with communication.

⚡ **Find your people:** You have got to surround yourself with people who get it. People love to judge others' parenting and it can be really hard if you're the only one with a neurodivergent kid, as you can feel so torn down. You'll find that your child naturally gravitates to other neurodivergent kids, so that's a great way in, or you can join an online community.

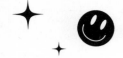

Getting a Diagnosis for Your Child

Heather Parks, the neurodivergent family coach we met in Chapter 11, helps families navigate the process of getting a diagnosis all the way through to finding support in social care systems and within education. She offers her advice for parents supporting their children through the diagnosis process ...

⚡ **It's going to be tough:** 'There are different systems in place across the country, and you're dealing with a lot of people who, unfortunately, you can't guarantee are going to listen to you and help you. A lot of my work involves dealing with families who are facing barrier after barrier, and they're not being believed or heard when it comes to seeking help and support for their child. They're going to schools or GPs (often the first port of call for a diagnosis) and having their concerns rejected to the extent that they start questioning themselves. You're simultaneously trying to clue yourself up to understand the new world of neurodiversity which you're landed and trying to navigate systems which are still largely operating from a deficit based model rather than the neurodiversity paradigm. It's a steep learning curve. Sadly many parents discover that the experts in whom they placed their trust have been unhelpful or even harmful. Parents often need support to see that they are the expert when it comes to their children.'

⚡ **Your love is so important:** 'So much more support out there is needed, but the best person to support your child is you. So it's vital you stay grounded in your own emotional experience and centred so you can be that calm support for your child. You're having to grapple with how you've been parented, as well as a traditional idea of what good parenting is. Extended family may be disbelieving and tell you that you "are being too soft, are letting them get away with too much or that you need to assert more control". There are so many harmful messages out there and there's a lot to face. I advise you to strip away society's "shoulds", the judgements, and connect with yourself and your child and what matters.'

⚡ **Watch out for people saying there's something 'wrong' with your child:** 'Doctors and teachers during this process might try to say your child just needs to change to fit into their environment, but – as we know – they're experiencing that environment in a totally different way to everyone else. It can be very easy for a parent to begin to believe what they're being told. This can happen even once a diagnosis has been reached, as a parent can think, "Ah, it's not just me being a bad parent, there's something wrong with my child and I can't do anything to help them; they need to learn to change." That's a really dangerous message, as you then start judging your child for not behaving or not trying hard enough or not being resilient enough, and they will pick up on that energy.'

⚡ **The process can bring up a lot of fear:** 'You're wanting to get them support and you're worried about what a diagnosis will mean for them in the long term. Will they make it through school? Will they be independent? We jump to the future instead of just being present and dealing with the current situation.'

The Part 3 Workbook
Navigating Neurodivergence

Chapter 9: School and University

1. Everyone's experience in education is different; if you have chosen to disclose with your school or university, do you feel like they've adequately supported you? Example: Have they actively taken the initiative to support you, or do you feel like you have been dismissed?

   ....

   ....

   ....

2. If you left education settings a long time ago, what comes up when you reflect on them (with the added context of neurodivergence)? Example: Perhaps you feel sad that you weren't offered the same opportunities that others were.

   ....

   ....

   ....

3. Have you managed to find any adjustments or accommodations that work for you? How has that impacted your experience? Example: You may now be able to work from home; how has this helped?

....
....
....

4. What could be changed to make the education environment/experience more neurodivergent-friendly for you personally? Example: Is it possible to have a quiet room away from the main area?

....
....
....

Chapter 10: Work

1. If you're someone who's struggled with the majority of workplace settings, do you feel like you might have internalised some of those negative experiences? Example: Do you feel like you struggle with confidence or feelings of inadequacy?

....

....

....

2. Things like productivity, speed and efficiency are valued in the society we live in, and it's often hard to separate yourself from those ideas. Do you think there are any signs of you still holding on to those standards in certain areas of your life? Example: Do you think you need to 'earn' time to relax? Do you tell yourself that you're 'failing' if you don't manage to make nutritious meals from scratch?

....

....

....

3. If you work, how neurodivergent-friendly would you say your workplace is? Can you think of anything that could be improved to make work easier for you? Example: Perhaps meetings could be set up in a way that relies less on taking on information verbally.

....

....

....

4. If we were all able to work for a reason that wasn't money, what would that look like for you? Example: Would you focus on creativity? Is there anything that you'd like to try/do more of that you don't feel works well alongside the fact that you have to earn an income?

....

....

....

5. What does 'success' really look like for you personally? Example: This may not look like a typical career path; it could be really understanding yourself or making a difference.

....

....

....

Chapter 11: Family and Friends

1. What's your relationship with your family like? Do you feel seen by them? Example: Are you close with your family? Has this changed at all over time?

....

....

....

2. Are there any honest truths you'd communicate with your family if you knew it wouldn't be received badly? Example: I felt sort of let down by you hiding my medical childhood diagnosis from me, and I felt like I would have known myself better if you hadn't withheld it from me.

    ....
    ....
    ....

3. If you're late-realised, do you hold any resentment towards anyone in your family for not noticing sooner? Or do you feel like they did what they could with what they had? (Both answers are valid – and might even change as your journey evolves.) Example: Maybe your parents used to joke about certain traits you displayed, and you feel annoyed they didn't take you more seriously.

    ....
    ....
    ....

4. Do you recognise any neurodivergent traits in other family members? Example: My mum's a keen info-dumper (and I love it).

    ....
    ....
    ....

5. Since your realisation, has your view on what a friendship should look like changed? Example: Perhaps you hold fewer expectations of people, or hold less anxiety towards maintaining friendships.

   ....

   ....

   ....

6. Is there anyone in your network that you feel particularly supported by? Example: This could also be an online friend or community!

   ....

   ....

   ....

7. If you've struggled with friendships in the past, do you now look at those difficulties differently with a little more understanding about the way you work? Example: Are you now able to communicate to your friends that certain environments are difficult for you?

   ....

   ....

   ....

Chapter 12: Relationships and Sex

1. Would you say you use sex or romantic relationships for excitement or stimulation? If so, do you carry any shame or regret around past experiences? Why do you think this is? Example: You may not have realised when you were younger that a lot of your sexual experiences were centred around impulsivity.

   ....

   ....

   ....

2. If you're in a relationship, would you say your partner is accepting and supportive of you being neurodivergent? If they aren't, is there any way you could communicate your needs in a different way? Is there anything you'd like them to research? Example: Perhaps their expectations of you are still above what you feel you can achieve.

   ....

   ....

   ....

3. If you experience sensory sensitivities, do you think this has an impact on sex for you (solo or otherwise)? Example: Perhaps you struggle with the feeling of certain sensations (e.g. massage, licking) that you feel you 'should' enjoy.

....

....

....

4. We all know that trauma and neurodivergence often go hand in hand. Do you think there might be any behaviours that you feel you need to pay closer attention to in order to maintain a healthy relationship? (FYI, this isn't a space for self-blame, but rather a place for balanced and gentle reflection.) Example: Perhaps due to past trauma you struggle with feelings of inadequacy that you sometimes project onto your partner.

....

....

....

5. What does the perfect partner/s look like for you? How would they be able to love and support you in the way you really need?

....

....

....

Chapter 13: Health, Fitness and Nutrition

1. What are your 'safe foods', if you have any?

....

....

....

2. Do you feel as though taking care of yourself feels unachievable? Are there any hacks that seem to make it easier? Example: Honestly, we'd be NOWHERE without adding in some novelty and romanticising the mundane.

....

....

....

3. If you could do any three things in the morning to give yourself the best chance at feeling good that day, what would they be? Example: Water before caffeine? A protein-heavy, pre-packaged snack? Listening to a soothing/grounding/upbeat playlist?

   ....
   ....
   ....

4. What is your relationship with exercise like? Does it feel like a chore? Is there any form of gentle exercise you enjoy? Example: Swimming or yoga.

   ....
   ....
   ....

5. Can you think of any way to make exercise more appealing if you're struggling with it? Example: A stroll combined with a phone call? A 10-minute bop to a delicious playlist?

   ....
   ....
   ....

Chapter 14: Life Admin

1. So many of us struggle with paying bills, making phone calls and arranging appointments. If you struggle with these things, how does it impact how you feel about yourself? What feelings come up when you put something off? Example: Putting off booking a doctor's appointment left us feeling like we were failing at being 'adults' but that's ridiculous, and it's okay to struggle. We're allowed to struggle and *ask for help*.

   ....

   ....

   ....

2. Do you feel as though there's anything in your life that you'd like to achieve but that feels unattainable for you? Example: Maybe you want to book a driving lesson, but never seem to get round to it. Perhaps you want to be self-employed, but the thought of managing the admin feels ... too much?

   ....

   ....

   ....

3. Have you tried a planner? (Only joking!) On a serious note, are there any ways you can make day-to-day life admin easier for yourself? Example: This could look like sharing a responsibility, doing these tasks on a body-doubling session (see page 295), or having someone else advocate for you when communicating with a healthcare professional.

    ....
    ....
    ....

4. Can you name **one** thing that you've been putting off that you would love to promise yourself you will do in the next week/month/year? Example: This could be as small as clearing up the glasses on your bedside table, or maybe you want to make that phone call to your doctor?

    ....
    ....
    ....

Chapter 15: Parenting

1. Can you think of anything you wish your parents could've done differently to support you as a child? Example: I wish my parents had had more patience with me.

   ....

   ....

   ....

2. If you're a parent, do you carry any shame around your parenting style? Or how easy/difficult you find it? Why do you think that is? Example: If you're a neurodivergent parent, do you struggle with how to navigate your own meltdowns or struggles to get things done? Do you think it might be because you're tied to standards that exclude you?

   ....

   ....

   ....

3. Is there anything you wish you knew about neurodivergence before you became a parent? Example: That I find loud noises extremely overstimulating, and that there ARE ways to help me manage my response to it.

....

....

....

4. After learning more comprehensively about neurodivergence, is there anything in particular that shifted your perspective when it came to either interacting with or parenting neurodivergent children? Example: Since we've learnt about how much energy *we*, as autistics spend on processing things, it's significantly shifted how I phrase questions, and the amount of time I give for them to be considered when talking to the neurodivergent littles in my life.

....

....

....

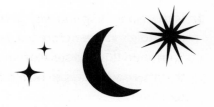

Conclusion

We're here! The end of the book ... but certainly not the end of our journey. As you can tell, we've done a hell of a lot of learning – about ourselves, others and the world – to get here and we don't think we'll ever stop doing that. We're not perfect – we never will be – we're just humans doing the best we can with our brains and this wild, surprising, often-not-built-for-us world.

We want to end this book on a high! To have a celebration of who we all are and how far we've all come. There are so many joyful things about being neurodivergent, things that make us wonderful, but (and by now you'll know we heart a disclaimer) we also want to begin the end by breaking down the whole 'superpower' thing. You know, how so many people love to say, 'Oh, being neurodivergent ... that's your superpower!' We don't want to dampen how anyone feels about their own brain. It's important for you to own your journey, and if saying you have a superpower helps you then go for it! But we do want the conversations around celebrating our spicy brains to come with a little nuance.

The thing about framing neurodiversity as a 'superpower' is that it tends to gloss over the hard parts – the fact that so many in our community are literally disabled in a world not designed for them. If people outside of that community think, 'Oh, it's a superpower,' that might mean they don't examine themselves, their workplaces, their friendships and parenting styles to see how they can adapt. The superpower thing places the burden on the individual to find that superpower within themselves, rather than putting the pressure on society to adapt. We need systemic change. A lot of our concerns around the superpower rhetoric is that it doesn't leave enough room for our struggles to be acknowledged. Often, the people we hear using it are very privileged, those who have a better time being neurodivergent or a parent to a neurodivergent child, because they have access to a lot more resources and support and all the other things that make life a bit easier. It might stop them recognising their own privilege and working to help and support others who are less fortunate.

What we love about ourselves!

Okay … now we've got that out of the way, we can celebrate! Because we're fucking awesome. So, we asked our community what they loved about being neurodivergent and this is what they had to say:

- ⚡ 'I am … me! Very weird thought, but it's always been my positive.'
- ⚡ 'Seeing through bullshit!'
- ⚡ 'I question everything!'

⚡ 'Creativity and a unique perspective.'

⚡ 'How much joy I can get from the little things and how big my feelings are in general.'

⚡ 'I'm never bored! My brain is a sparkly party compared to other people's!'

⚡ 'The energy and creative highs (the lows ... less so).'

⚡ 'Feeling deep joy and wonder at beautiful things, being hyperlexic [being able to read very early] and loving language.'

⚡ 'I'm a multi-tasking demon who loves change and solving problems.'

⚡ 'My super-high empathy and how that makes me care so much for other people.'

⚡ 'Endless curiosity.'

⚡ 'I am genuinely the funniest person I know.'

⚡ 'I'm hellbent on changing the world in the name of justice!'

⚡ 'Seeing all the patterns and connections, noticing the details.'

⚡ 'Standing up for what is right! No matter the social consequences for myself!'

⚡ 'We often have the biggest personalities and hearts.'

⚡ 'How I problem-solve and think so creatively.'

⚡ 'I love that I hyperfocus.'

⚡ 'The way I listen to music and can hear every instrument like I'm floating.'

⚡ 'My deep capacity to love.'

⚡ 'Seeing the best in everyone.'

Awww! That's made us feel all warm and fuzzy. It's also really helped us to pinpoint what we love about being neurodivergent: a task, we must admit, we struggled with at first. Not because we don't love ourselves, but because our experiences are so wrapped up in being individuals, it's hard to pinpoint what's neurodiversity, what's trauma and what's just ... us! We also found that our brains naturally (because of this silly capitalist world we live in) headed towards what makes us useful (which we don't want to focus on; we're not robots!), but with a little help from each other this is what we decided ...

JESS: I can say confidently that I'm an extremely attentive friend to the right people. I'm passionate, keen to see people for who they are, and give them what they need. I hope that my friendship brings comfort and validation. If those around me are deserving of these parts of myself, they will get them in abundance. I've definitely been the 'personality hire' of a few workplaces, where a lack of understanding of my needs meant I struggled with the day-to-day tasks of the job, but I was likely given leniency as I brought a 'vibrant' energy to the office.

I love the fact that I've been told by my friends that they feel comfortable being themselves around me. Given my own experience with fluctuating energy levels, so many of my relationships are now built on a mutual understanding that energy for socialising is never assumed. I'd like to think that I take that same awareness of energy levels into all of my interactions, and I can only hope that means my friendship feels like a safe, cosy place for the people I care about. I'd say this might also be the reason that as a community, we're some of the least judgemental people around. It allows you such freedom to be yourself.

MIA: I like my slight obsessiveness, how I can pull things apart and look at them in a different way. That's a work one, and I don't want my ability to hyperfocus to be abused, but when I'm in the mode it's a wonderful feeling. I also apply that way of thinking to my humour; it's dry and dark. I can evaluate situations and then plainly take the piss out of them. It's fun. We also both have such empathy. I feel like we have the same brain at times. There's no expectation from each other, as there has been with other friends. We've known each other for 10 years and I think we've sent three birthday cards in that time. We're aware of the demands we place on each other, and we tread carefully and support each other in a way that's truly needed – that isn't just, 'Oh, do you need a hug?' Our brains see what's actually needed and then we offer that.

Autistic people can be so brilliantly straight-forward; there's never any of that anxiety of reading between the lines and trying to figure out where you stand. We come up with our opinions and do our own research. We've had to actively do the opposite of what society is asking of us so many times, because we can't manage or maintain it, so it's nice to have a community of people who are encouraging and supportive of you going against the grain and putting your wellbeing first.

Before We Reach the Very End … (Sob!)

We've said it throughout the book, but we just want to make ourselves absolutely clear on a couple of things: the first is privilege. We're so aware that we are writing this book from a privileged position, and it's always been vitally important to us to actively listen to and learn from other people in our community, particularly those who are marginalised. This isn't just us paying lip service; we'd hate for anyone to think we're just saying this to cover our own backs. Through our platform, and wherever possible, **we are trying to champion other voices and people**.

Also, we'd like to point out that we're not doctors or professionals (ha – in case you hadn't noticed!); we're just here, sharing our experiences, hoping they can help. We want all of you to go on your own journey, to feel empowered to do your own research and, whether it's through self-realisation or a diagnosis, to come to a place where you feel happy in yourself and with who you are. Don't feel you have to copy everything we've said or done word for word – this is your glorious path!

A Final Word from Us!

It's been a **ride**, and we know we've spoken about some pretty heavy stuff, which – if you are at the beginning of your journey – might make you want to stick your fingers in your ears and scream, 'No, I don't want to do that. Let me be!' But we really want to emphasise just how transformative this has all been for us. It's utterly surreal to live a life that feels this much easier and softer than we'd ever imagined possible.

We used to feel like time didn't belong to us. That peace didn't belong to us. Our lives were full of dread and anxiety. We were staying in relationships, jobs, friendships that weren't serving us, and which we couldn't see a way out of. We stayed because our confidence was so low, but also because we couldn't **see** why they weren't serving us, why we were working so hard and seeing no reward ...

So how have we got to this place where we feel so much joy? Where we feel so much like our true selves? Where we've freed ourselves from (most of) the shit that was leaving us deeply miserable? We didn't believe this state of mind existed, never mind that we might actually get here.

We haven't suppressed who we are. **We haven't tried to fit in.** We haven't tried to avoid the gritty, grief-filled parts. We squash that voice in our head that tells us our experiences aren't valid and we're gentle with ourselves when we mess up. We're not holding ourselves to the same unobtainable standards we were before.

We've all been encouraged, pretty much from the get-go, to suppress our needs, either because they've been invalidated or because we've felt embarrassed to even voice them in the first place. But we're telling you, as loudly as we possibly can, that getting to know your own needs is the best way to honour them. We deserve to prioritise ourselves unapologetically. There have been so many times in our lives when we haven't been able to get what we need because we didn't even know what the problem was. There were so many situations where we didn't feel comfortable and didn't want to do certain things, and we didn't realise how much that affected us.

This led to us making mistakes and seeking validation in all the wrong places. Staying in situations that made us deeply unhappy. We're learning to forgive ourselves, and we want you to be able to do that, too. Accepting who you are is also about accepting your fuck-ups. Knowing that you are doing, and have done, the best you can, with what you have at the time. Make room for those mistakes; they are learning moments.

As for that grief? Those truly awful times? They were real. They were hard. We got through them, and so will you. Grief is a powerful thing. We don't expect to be able to erase it; instead, we carry it with us. We're open about it in the most vulnerable way – and that helps us.

So, here's our manifesto: what we will keep doing, and what we want you to do as well ... Repeat after us:

- ⚡ We won't feel apologetic for asking for what we need.
- ⚡ We will advocate for ourselves, saying, 'This is what we respect, and we need you to respect that, too.'
- ⚡ We will carry our grief, knowing that it's real and powerful.
- ⚡ We will forgive ourselves. Constantly. Know that our mistakes are our learnings.
- ⚡ We will tell people how we need to be loved.
- ⚡ We will celebrate the little things – the washing being done and hung up, the days we made it out of bed.
- ⚡ We won't let our focus on what's coming next take away from where we're at now.
- ⚡ We will keep trying.
- ⚡ We will keep helping each other and our community.
- ⚡ We will not shame ourselves for where we're at.
- ⚡ We will continue to be human and (messy) and beautiful.
- ⚡ We know that there's nothing disordered about us.

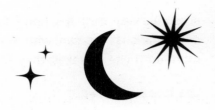

Notes

Introduction

1. 'New Guidance: Neurodiversity in the Workplace', British Dyslexia Association (20 March 2019): www.bdadyslexia.org.uk/news/new-guidance-neurodiversity-in-the-workplace
2. Autism Statistics, April 2021 to Match 2022, NHS Digital: https://digital.nhs.uk/data-and-information/publications/statistical/autism-statistics/april-2021-to-march-2022

Chapter 2 – What Is Neurodivergence?

1. Nicole Baumer and Julia Frueh, 'What is neurodiversity?', **Harvard Health Publishing** (23 November 2021): www.health.harvard.edu/blog/what-is-neurodiversity-202111232645
2. 'What is autism?', National Autistic Society: www.autism.org.uk/advice-and-guidance/what-is-autism
3. 'Attention deficit hyperactivity disorder', NHS: https://www.nhs.uk/conditions/attention-deficit-hyperactivity-disorder-adhd/
4. 'Attention deficit hyperactivity disorder: How common is it?' National Institute for Health and Care Excellence (revised November 2022): https://cks.nice.org.uk/topics/attention-deficit-hyperactivity-disorder/background-information/prevalence/

5. Ayesha Khan, 'Yes, we're all a little neurodivergent', Woke Scientist Substack (21 April 2022): https://wokescientist.substack.com/p/yes-were-all-a-little-neurodivergent

Chapter 3 – Key Signs

1. 'Symptoms: Attention deficit hyperactivity disorder', NHS: www.nhs.uk/conditions/attention-deficit-hyperactivity-disorder-adhd/symptoms/
2. 'Attention deficit hyperactivity disorder (ADHD)', NHSinform.scot
3. 'Signs of autism in adults', NHS: www.nhs.uk/conditions/autism/signs/adults/
4. 'Stimming', National Autistic Society: www.autism.org.uk/advice-and-guidance/topics/behaviour/stimming
5. 'Social model of disability', Scope: www.scope.org.uk/about-us/social-model-of-disability/

Chapter 4 – Why Are Autism and ADHD So Underdiagnosed?

1. Autism Statistics, April 2021 to Match 2022, NHS Digital: https://digital.nhs.uk/data-and-information/publications/statistical/autism-statistics/april-2021-to-march-2022
2. 'Autism Statistics and Facts', Autism Speaks: www.autismspeaks.org/autism-statistics-asd
3. Ibid.
4. Ibid.
5. Ibid.
6. Robert McCrossin, 'Finding the True Number of Females with Autistic Spectrum Disorder by Estimating the Biases in Initial Recognition and Clinical Diagnosis', **Children** (Basel), 9: 2 (17 February 2022), 272: https://pubmed.ncbi.nlm.nih.gov/35204992/
7. Francesca Happé, 'Finding the female face of autism', The Academy of Medical Sciences (23 May 2018): https://acmedsci.ac.uk/more/news/finding-the-female-face-of-autism
8. Ibid.

9. 'Mental Health Among Autistic LGBTQ Youth', The Trevor Project (29 April 2022): www.thetrevorproject.org/research-briefs/mental-health-among-autistic-lgbtq-youth-apr-2022/

10. Nancy Doyle, 'ADHD Crisis in the UK: Under diagnosed, Lacking Support and Stigmatized', **Forbes** (14 Jan 2022): https://www.forbes.com/sites/drnancydoyle/2022/01/14/adhd-crisis-in-the-uk-under-diagnosed-lacking-support-and-stigmatized/?sh=78bd1d2a96f4

11. Florence Mowlem, 'Using an epidemiological approach to investigate sex differences in the manifestation of ADHD in youth and adulthood', King's College London (PhD thesis, 2018): https://kclpure.kcl.ac.uk/portal/files/106425259/2019_Mowlem_Florence_1414261_ethesis.pdf

12. Florence Mowlem et al., 'Do different factors influence whether girls versus boys meet ADHD diagnostic criteria? Sex differences among children with high ADHD symptoms', **Psychiatry Research**, 272 (February 2019), 765–773: www.sciencedirect.com/science/article/pii/S0165178118317347#!

13. Florence Mowlem et al., 'Sex differences in predicting ADHD clinical diagnosis and pharmacological treatment', **European Child & Adolescent Psychiatry**, 28 (2019), 481–489: https://link.springer.com/article/10.1007/s00787-018-1211-3

14. Devon Frye, 'The Children Left Behind', **Additude** (31 March 2022): https://www.additudemag.com/race-and-adhd-how-people-of-color-get-left-behind/

15. 'Attention-deficit/hyperactivity disorder and its comorbidities in women and girls: an evolving picture', Curr Psychiatry Rep., 2008 Oct;10(5):419-23. doi: 10.1007/s11920-008-0067-5.

16. www.instagram.com/tv/CLmqw2yjuLE/?igshid=MzRlODBiNWFlZA%3D%3D

17. Gray Atherton et al., 'Autism through the ages: A mixed methods approach to understanding how age and age of diagnosis affect quality of life', **Journal of Autism and Developmental Disorders**, 52 (2022), 3639–3654: https://doi.org/10.1007/s10803-021-05235-x

18. Ibid.

19. 'Signs and symptoms: Suicide and autism', Autistica: www.autistica.org.uk/what-is-autism/signs-and-symptoms/suicide-and-autism

20. 'Mental Health Among Autistic LGBTQ Youth', The Trevor Project: www.thetrevorproject.org/research-briefs/mental-health-among-autistic-lgbtq-youth-apr-2022/

21. 'Signs and symptoms: Suicide and autism', Autistica: www.autistica.org.uk/what-is-autism/signs-and-symptoms/suicide-and-autism

22. Alaa M. Hamed et al., 'Why the Diagnosis of Attention Deficit Hyperactivity Disorder Matters', **Frontiers in Psychiatry**, 6 (26 November 2015), 168: www.ncbi.nlm.nih.gov/pmc/articles/PMC4659921/

23. Kenneth Man et al., 'Attention deficit hyperactivity disorder, physical abuse and methylphenidate treatment in children', **Nature Mental Health**, 1 (2023), 66–75: https://doi.org/10.1038/s44220-022-00008-6

24. Courtney Zulauf, 'The Complicated Relationship Between Attention Deficit/Hyperactivity Disorder and Substance Use Disorders', **Current Psychiatry Reports**, 16: 3 (March 2014), 436: doi: 10.1007/s11920-013-0436-6

25. Morénike Giwa Onaiwu, '"They Don't Know, Don't Show, or Don't Care": Autism's White Privilege Problem', **Autism in Adulthood** (December 2020), 270–272: http://doi.org/10.1089/aut.2020.0077

26. Ibid.

27. 'I am a Black Caribbean woman with ADHD. No one believes me.', iampayingattention.co.uk

28. Autism Statistics, April 2021 to Match 2022, NHS Digital: https://digital.nhs.uk/data-and-information/publications/statistical/autism-statistics/april-2021-to-march-2022

Chapter 5 – Do You Need a Diagnosis?

1. 'What happens during an autism assessment', www.nhs.uk
2. 'Recognising autism in girls within the education context: reflecting on the internal presentation and the diagnostic criteria', *Irish Educational Studies*, doi: 10.1080/03323315.2023.2260371
3. 'What happens during an autism assessment', NHS: www.nhs.uk/conditions/autism/getting-diagnosed/assessments
4. 'Diagnosis: Attention deficit hyperactivity disorder (ADHD)', nhs.uk
5. 'Treatments that are not recommended for autism', NHS: www.nhs.uk/conditions/autism/autism-and-everyday-life/treatments-that-are-not-recommended-for-autism/
6. Nicholas Sheppard, 'The cruelty of Jacinda Ardern's immigration policy?' **Spectator** (28 April 2022): www.spectator.co.uk/article/does-jacinda-ardern-practise-what-she-preaches-about-kindness/
7. James Tapper, 'Fury at "do not resuscitate" notices given to Covid patients with learning disabilities', **Guardian** (13 February 2021): www.theguardian.com/world/2021/feb/13/new-do-not-resuscitate-orders-imposed-on-covid-19-patients-with-learning-difficulties

Chapter 6 – To Mask or Not to Mask?

1. Dr Hannah Belcher, 'Autistic people and masking', National Autistic Society (7 July 2022): www.autism.org.uk/advice-and-guidance/professional-practice/autistic-masking
2. Louise Bradley et al., 'Autistic Adults' Experiences of Camouflaging and Its Perceived Impact on Mental Health', **Autism Adulthood**, 3: 4 (1 December 2021), 320–329: doi: 10.1089/aut.2020.0071; Laura Hull et al., 'Development and Validation of the Camouflaging Autistic Traits Questionnaire (CAT-Q)', **Journal of Autism and Developmental Disorders**, 49: 3 (March 2019), 819–833: doi: 10.1007/s10803-018-3792-6
3. Sarah Cassidy et al., 'Risk markers for suicidality in autistic adults', **Molecular Autism**, 9: 42 (2018): https://doi.org/10.1186/s13229-018-0226-4

4. James Buehler, 'Racial/Ethnic Disparities in the Use of Lethal Force by US Police, 2010–2014', **American Journal of Public Health**, 107 (2017), 295–297: https://doi.org/10.2105/AJPH.2016.303575

5. K.L. Curry et al., 'Training criminal justice personnel to recognize offenders with disabilities', **OSERS News in Print**, 5: 3 (1993), 4–8: https://www.ojp.gov/pdffiles1/Digitization/142440NCJRS.pdf

6. Mental Health Act Statistics, Annual Figures 2021–22, NHS Digital: https://digital.nhs.uk/data-and-information/publications/statistical/mental-health-act-statistics-annual-figures/2021-22-annual-figures

Chapter 7 – Grief and Burnout

1. 'The Five Stages of Grief: An Examination of the Kubler-Ross Model', Psycom (7 June 2022): https://www.psycom.net/stages-of-grief

2. Szu-Ching Shen et al., 'Incidence, risk, and associated factors of depression in adults with physical and sensory disabilities: A nationwide population-based study', **PLoS One**, 12: 3 (31 March 2017), e0175141: doi: 10.1371/journal.pone.0175141

3. Samuel Arnold et al., 'Confirming the nature of autistic burnout', **Autism**, 0: 0 (2023): https://doi.org/10.1177/13623613221147410

Chapter 8 – Dealing with the Fallout

1. Nicole LePera, **How to Do the Work** (Orion Spring, 2021)

2. Freya Rumball et al., 'Experience of Trauma and PTSD Symptoms in Autistic Adults: Risk of PTSD Development Following DSM-5 and Non-DSM-5 Traumatic Life Events', **Autism Research**, 13: 12 (December 2020), 2122–2132. doi: 10.1002/aur.2306; Freya Rumball et al., 'Heightened risk of posttraumatic stress disorder in adults with autism spectrum disorder: The role of cumulative trauma and memory deficits', **Research in Developmental Disabilities**, 110 (March 2021), 103848: https://doi.org/10.1016/j.ridd.2020.103848; Nirit Haruvi-Lamdan et al., 'Autism Spectrum Disorder and Post-Traumatic Stress Disorder: An unexplored co-occurrence of

conditions', **Autism**, 24: 4 (May 2020), 884–898. doi:
10.1177/1362361320912143

3. Dr Freya Rumball, 'Post-traumatic stress disorder in autistic
people', National Autistic Society (30 March 2022): https://www.
autism.org.uk/advice-and-guidance/professional-practice/ptsd-
autism

Chapter 9 – School and University

1. 'Autism at University – being an autistic student', University of
Bristol (9 December 2020): https://www.bristol.ac.uk/blackwell/
news/2020/autism-at-university--being-an-autistic-student.html;
Eilidh Cage and Jack Howes, 'Dropping out and moving on: A
qualitative study of autistic people's experiences of university',
Autism, 24: 7 (2020), 1664–1675: https://doi.
org/10.1177/1362361320918750

2. Jenny Shaw and Freya Selman, 'An Asset, Not a Problem: Meeting
the Needs of Neurodivergent Students', Unite Students (2023):
https://www.unitegroup.com/neurodivergent-students-report

Chapter 10 – Work

1. 'Neurodivergent employees impacted by lack of training and
support in the workplace', City & Guilds (10 March 2023): www.
cityandguilds.com/news/march-2023/neurodivergent-employees-
impacted-by-lack-of-training-and-support-in-the-workplace

2. 'Employment in the UK: July 2023', Office for National Statistics:
https://www.ons.gov.uk/employmentandlabourmarket/
peopleinwork/employmentandemployeetypes/bulletins/
employmentintheuk/july2023

3. 'Asking your employer for changes to help you if you're disabled',
Citizens Advice: https://www.citizensadvice.org.uk/work/
discrimination-at-work/discrimination-at-work/taking-action/
asking-your-employer-for-changes-to-help-if-youre-disabled/

4. 'Why persistence matters more to ADHD than consistency', adhd-
couple.com

5. '7 Benefits of Employing Autistic Individuals', Enna: https://enna. org/7-benefits-of-employing-autistic-individuals

6. Kerry Chillemi, 'Understanding ADHD and Autistic Burnout Within the Workplace', **Psychology Today** (2 July 2022): https://www. psychologytoday.com/gb/blog/functional-legacy-mindset/202207/ understanding-adhd-and-autistic-burnout-within-the-workplace

Chapter 12 – Relationships and Sex

1. Devon Price, 'No, Mental Illness Isn't "Caused" by Chemicals in the Brain', Medium (16 June 2021): https://devonprice.medium.com/ no-mental-illness-isnt-caused-by-chemicals-in-the-brain- 1b01d6808871

2. John Anderson, 'LGBTQIA+ and neurodiversity: the links between neurodivergence and being LGBTQ+', The Brain Charity (23 December 2022): https://www.thebraincharity.org.uk/lgbtqia- neurodiversity-neurodivergent-lgbtq/#

3. Varun Warrier et al., 'Elevated rates of autism, other neurodevelopmental and psychiatric diagnoses, and autistic traits in transgender and gender-diverse individuals', **Nature Communications**, 11 (2020), 3959: https://doi.org/10.1038/s41467- 020-17794-1

4. Dr Nick Walker, **Neuroqueer Heresies: Notes on the Neurodiversity Paradigm, Autistic Empowerment, and Postnormal Possibilities** (Autonomous Press, 2021); Neuroqueer: The Writings of Dr Nick Walker: https://neuroqueer.com/ neuroqueer-an-introduction/

Chapter 13 – Health, Fitness and Nutrition

1. 'Experiences of being in hospital for people with a learning disability', Care Quality Commission (3 November 2022): https:// www.cqc.org.uk/publication/experiences-being-hospital-people- learning-disability-and-autistic-people/report

2. Ulrica Nilsson, 'Soothing music can increase oxytocin levels during bed rest after open-heart surgery: a randomised control trial',

Journal of Clinical Nursing, 18: 15 (August 2009), 2153–61. doi: 10.1111/j.1365-2702.2008.02718.x; Jill Suttie, 'Four Ways Music Strengthens Social Bonds', **Greater Good Magazine** (15 January 2015): https://greatergood.berkeley.edu/article/item/four_ways_music_strengthens_social_bonds

3. Brett Milano, 'Probing the Sleep-deprived Brain', **Harvard Gazette** (30 March 2018): https://news.harvard.edu/gazette/story/2018/03/harvard-talk-probes-sleep-deprived-brain

4. Preeti Devnani and Anaita Hegde, 'Autism and sleep disorders', **Journal of Pediatric Neurosciences**, 10: 4 (2015), 304–7: doi: 10.4103/1817-1745.174438

5. Emma Beddington, 'The seven types of rest: I spent a week trying them all. Could they help end my exhaustion?' **Guardian** (25 November 2021): https://www.theguardian.com/lifeandstyle/2021/nov/25/the-seven-types-of-rest-i-spent-a-week-trying-them-all-could-they-help-end-my-exhaustion; Saundra Dalton-Smith, **Sacred Rest: Recover Your Life, Renew Your Energy, Restore Your Sanity** (FaithWords, 2017)

6. Luke Curtis and Kalpana Patel, 'Nutritional and environmental approaches to preventing and treating autism and attention deficit hyperactivity disorder (ADHD): a review', **Journal of Alternative and Complementary Medicine**, 14: 1 (January–February 2008), 79–85: doi: 10.1089/acm.2007.0610

7. Beat Eating Disorders: https://www.beateatingdisorders.org.uk/

8. Noriko Numata et al., 'Associations between autism spectrum disorder and eating disorders with and without self-induced vomiting: an empirical study', **Journal of Eating Disorders**, 9(1): 5 (6 January 2021): doi: 10.1186/s40337-020-00359-4

9. Bruno Nazar et al., 'The risk of eating disorders comorbid with attention-deficit/hyperactivity disorder: A systematic review and meta-analysis', **International Journal of Eating Disorders**, 49: 12 (December 2016), 1045–1057: doi: 10.1002/eat.22643.https://pubmed.ncbi.nlm.nih.gov/27859581/

10. Patty Onderko, 'What's the Link Between ADHD and Eating Disorders?' HealthCentral (updated 13 September 2022): www.healthcentral.com/article/the-link-between-adhd-and-eating-disorders
11. Kathrin Nickel et al., 'Systematic Review: Overlap Between Eating, Autism Spectrum, and Attention-Deficit/Hyperactivity Disorder', **Frontiers in Psychiatry**, 10 (10 October 2019): https://doi.org/10.3389/fpsyt.2019.00708

Chapter 14 – Life Admin

1. 'How Does ADHA Affect Executive Function?' The ADHD Centre (16 November 2022): https://www.adhdcentre.co.uk/how-does-adhd-affect-executive-function/
2. 'The ADHD Interest-Based Nervous System', MedCircle (26 September 2022): https://medcircle.com/articles/adhd-interest-based-nervous-system/

Chapter 15 – Parenting

1. Bethan Staton, 'Thousands of children aren't turning up to school post-lockdown. Why?' **Financial Times** (26 October 2022): www.ft.com/content/e9c632bf-5f42-4e83-a0b8-ea14b8bb8aa5

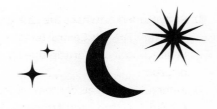

Resources

It's not only us screaming into the internet about why we ND folk matter. These accounts and communities are also doing some incredible work to make us late-diagnosed or late-realised folk feel seen. Our monotropic minds want to tell you every single tiny thing about why we love these creators, but we're going to try to stick to a few words!

Wemzy @aqotas A parent who shows her followers affirming ways to raise autistic children. She also runs an amazing sensory toy kit business called @aqotassensorytoys

@adhdbabes Founded by Vivienne Isebor @vvnsings. A support group for Black women and Black non-binary folk of African and Caribbean descent with ADHD.

Rach Idowu @adultingadhd A good friend of ours, Rach created a gorgeous set of ADHD flashcards showing different traits, examples and top tips. She also talks about intersectionality and normalising the reality of life with ADHD.

Sonny Jane Wise @livedexperienceeducator Sonny is a neurodivergent, disabled and queer creator who challenges the idea that having ADHD or autism is a disorder and centres variation and diversity as normal parts of human existence.

Tiffany L. Hammond @fidgets.and.fries A bestselling children's author (her beautiful book is called **A Day with No Words** (Wheat Penny Press, 2023), inspired by her non-speaking son) who talks about the nuances of being Black and autistic and explains that we won't all experience our diagnoses in the same way.

René Brooks @blackgirllostkeys One of the first people we started following when we were dipping our toes into the neurodivergent pool on Twitter, René has a tonne of blog posts with helpful tips (plus she offers coaching services!).

Dr Ayesha Khan @wokescientist When it comes to looking at neurodiversity through a community-focused, anti-capitalist lens, we're truly in awe of Ayesha, who is also the writer of an incredible newsletter called Cosmic Anarchy.

Jesse Meadows @jessethesluggish Jesse critiques some of the language and theories within the neurodivergent community – if you're anything like us, you'll find her perspectives refreshing as hell.

Morgan Harper Nichols @morganharpernichols An autistic ADHDer who happens to create some of the most aesthetically beautiful, soothing posts we've ever seen – 10/10 recommend if you want to feel a bit more at ease about existing.

Ingri @adhd_couple Practical tips, awareness and lots of information, all wrapped up in deliciously presented illustrations.

Dr Devon Price @drdevonprice Author Dr Devon Price takes a logical approach to debunking a lot of the rhetoric when it comes to neurodivergence. Honestly? We feel a lot freer having heard it.

Kirsti Hadley @generationalalphabet A late-realised AuDHDer and mother of an ND child, Kirsti, who you heard from in Chapter 15, is a loud advocate and regularly partakes in campaigns for accessible, inclusive education settings.

Alexis Lee @stylemesunday We couldn't love Alexis more. She's a dyslexic ADHDer who offers plenty of insightful, brutally honest insights as she heals. She also wrote a fantastic book, **Feeling Myself** (Vermillion, 2022), about finding sexual freedom.

Yasmin Johal @yasminjohalx An incredibly well-dressed autistic parent to an autistic child, who regularly graces our feed with doses of the autistic joy we all need.

Tiffany @nigh.functioning.autism An overwhelmingly great educator, ND parent to ND children, and user of and advocate for alternative communication methods.

Lou @neurodivergent_lou Lou's posts are super informative, expertly written and easy to digest; they tick all the boxes when it comes to validation and education about all things autism.

Charlie Clement @charliclement_ A truly GORGEOUS mix of recommendations, education and empowerment relating to disability and identity.

Ellen Jones @ellen_jones Ellen is an educator and speaker who is good at too many things for us to list, but take it from us, your feed will be better with this impressive and honest human in it.

Acknowledgements

Mia

To Ols who has (literally) financed, fuelled and encouraged me on this journey. Thanks for believing in me and hyping me up in that awkward business start-up stage when everyone else thought it was another 'phase' of mine. Thanks for the 197 cups of coffee and dragging me out of bed, 293 sandwiches when I am working through lunch and the regular glasses of wine you bring me while I am aggressively hyper-focusing at 9pm. Thanks for enduring the mood swings and outbursts while I was figuring out what the fuck was going on in my brain and having super human patience (a trait I envy). I love you endlessly.

To Mama and Colin, the best cheerleaders who have supported me emotionally, financially and physically through the ugliest times (like really ugly, the times when only your parents could love you). Thank you for taking me all the way back and forth from university even though I never learnt anything, and for being there to celebrate, cry and scream. Thank you for believing in our (little) business; your belief and trust in what we could achieve has been monumental in getting me to where I am today. Finally, thanks Mama for always being the ultimate badass role model for me, your creativity, ambition (and impulsivity) inspire me every day.

To my sister, we are more alike than we will ever know and for that reason drive each other up the wall! Please know I am always here and I am really proud of everything you have achieved.

To Grandma and Grandad, thank you for always offering a safe place for me to come and stay, drink tea, play badminton, dress up, play games and eat the best chips in the world.

Jess

There are many people who've been a part of the journey I speak of in this book – some are still in my life, and some aren't. While I'm of course deeply, deeply appreciative of the people who've managed to get me through the rough times, for me, writing a list of names feels a little too restrictive – maybe not quite encapsulating **exactly** what got me here.

While I'm not a cold-hearted witch and will continue to remind those who I think need to hear it how grateful I am, let me instead use this space to articulate how much having people in my life who make me feel safe to be myself has changed **everything**.

Thank you for learning with me, and for reminding me with actions that superficial relationships will never be for me. Your love, wisdom, respect and perspective is something I'll never take for granted, and I'm not sure I'd be here without it.

Thank you to the online community who we've learned from, your wisdom, stories, heartfelt messages and comments have all made me feel more at home within myself than I've ever done before.

Oh, and a quick shout out to the people who were awful. Thank you for giving me no choice but to switch things up, ditch the toxicity, and eventually find myself here, it feels extra delicious.

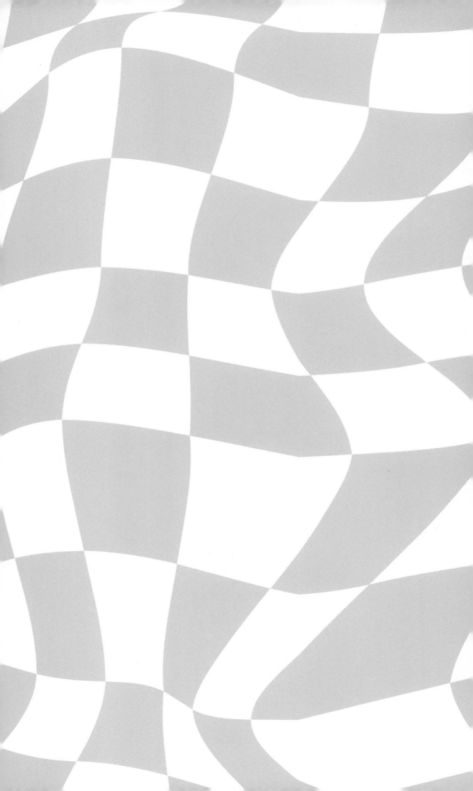